BECOMING OVARY JONES

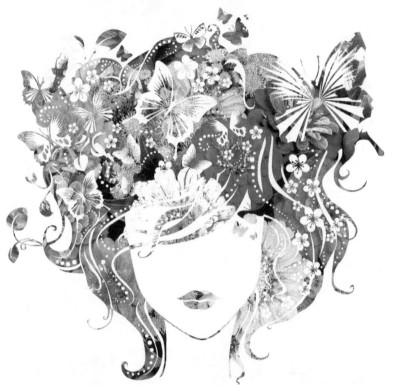

BECOMING
OVARY
JONES

How to Fight Cancer Without Losing Your Mind

MELANIE HOLSCHER

HOUNDSTOOTH
PRESS

BECOMING OVARY JONES

How to Fight Cancer Without Losing Your Mind

ISBN   978-1-5445-1645-5 *Hardcover*

      978-1-5445-1644-8 *Paperback*

      978-1-5445-1643-1 *Ebook*

To all Ovary Jones warriors...

May we find a cure.

Until then, may we find strength through cancer.

CONTENTS

ACKNOWLEDGMENTS

Please don't try to fight cancer alone. Let this natural disaster bring you closer to your family and friends. It would be impossible for me to acknowledge all the people who have had a big impact on my life. Through this storm, there were many who held the umbrella for me while I was down, and there were some who danced with me in the rain.

Nick, Caleb, Mackenzie, and Paisley Holscher, Scott Brewer, and my parents Chuck and Donna—love is motivating.

In addition to my incredible family, I'd like to thank:

Dr. Eirwen Miller, Dr. Sarah Miller, and the entire Allegheny Health Network oncology team, and Gregory S. Willis, DO, Pinnacle Health Oncologist

Coaches are amazing, and these cherished saints led me through so much:

Angie Moss

Rebecca Swanson

Katie Hasson

Jay Jones

Dana Potthoff

When we find meaningful work, we are truly blessed. Thank you for the work that you do and the inspiration through this journey:

Dustin and Kyah Hillis

Van Alford (Ron Alford)

Shannon Simon

Christa Acevedo

Ron and Kittie Barrow

Dave and Emmie Brown

Gena Parker

Rebecca Goldsberry

Karla Lewis

Christina Gradillas

Brent Widman

Teej Cummings

Joe Noonan

Clark Short

Leslie Montgomery

Rob and Julie Novak

Vince Coyle

Kacy Discher

Bonnie Diver

Hair Peace Charities

The Mary Moore Foundation—Tina Logan

Our inner circle knows us best. Thanks to these people for sticking with me through thick and thin:

Tom Rowden

Julie Biggs

Lori Sadler

Amy Porter Greco

Dr. Arif Mohamed

Beth Parson

Jackie Stanton

Susan Miller

Tabitha Laine

Paul Swann

Finally, thanks to these men for studying and shining a light on the Word of God:

Joe Pisano

Perry Lemmons

INTRODUCTION

Where are you right now with your cancer diagnosis? Maybe you found this book shortly after you consulted with your doctor, and it doesn't even seem real yet. Perhaps you've had some time to absorb the news, and you are figuring out a plan. It is a lot to take in. Hearing the "C" word was as disappointing to me as I'm sure it was for you. Whatever you are feeling right now is okay. It's understandable. Go ahead and feel it. Give yourself permission to express your feelings. Close the door and have a good cry or scream some bad words. This isn't a "suck it up, buttercup" moment. As a society, I think we sweep things under the rug way too much. We expect people to leave their emotions at home as if that's possible. We were created with emotions. In fact, emotions are a gift. I understand the emotions you are feeling now are neither pleasant nor fun, but you can't ignore them. Recognize and acknowledge them. Try to identify and name them. Fear.

Anger. Disgust. Confusion. Sadness. I found writing down exactly what I was feeling helped me accept my diagnosis. I also found I needed to do it more than once. It is a process. Sometimes I had friends that I could vent to, but often it was just me alone with an innocent sheet of paper when I poured out my heart.

Right now, there is a lot of uncertainty. The future looks blurry. When embarking on a journey, usually we map out our course and set out with confidence, knowing if we follow the plan, we will arrive safely at our destination. Once you and your doctors start to map out your cancer journey, you quickly realize the path has many twists and turns. It requires flexibility and problem solving. Even if you typically enjoy spontaneity, the seriousness of the situation is sobering. This isn't an experience you signed up for. It was chosen for you.

THE WAITING GAME

One of the most frustrating and downright maddening things about fighting cancer is all of the waiting. Waiting in the waiting room. Waiting in various sci-fi devices (MRIs, CAT scans, Radiation tables). Waiting for test results. Waiting for side effects to subside. Waiting between treatments. Waiting. Waiting. Waiting. I'm willing to bet the waiting is even challenging for the most patient among us, although I wouldn't know because I've never been known for my patience.

Becoming Ovary Jones: How to Fight Cancer without Losing Your Mind will help. You are not alone. We've all been there. Many of us will be there again. I truly believe this journey will strengthen you. You can actually become a better version of yourself through your cancer adventure. It all comes down to one very important decision that you have to make. Are you going to give cancer all the power, or are you going to use cancer as a tool for your betterment?

Welcome to the club. Regardless of how you choose to respond to your diagnosis, we welcome you with open arms and accept you just as you are. You happen to have cancer. Perhaps you have friends and family members who have or had cancer, too. Maybe you personally don't know anybody who has been in this ring. It won't be long, and you will know a lot of brave cancer warriors. Everybody always asks me about this Ovary Jones club. Who is Ovary Jones anyway? That's an interesting story actually.

Unfortunately, I didn't realize I had cancer until it was pretty bad. I never asked about staging until recently, but I knew it was bad. They admitted me into the hospital immediately. It turned out I had a tumor the size of a grapefruit that was growing quickly in my abdomen. I had no idea it was there. Apparently, all of my organs mind their own business. You would think one of them would have sent a message to my brain alerting me to the fact there was a visitor in there. It turns out my organs are nonconfrontational, and this giant tumor was a bully that had started choking out my spinal column. That's when I started to notice I had a problem.

My situation seemed awfully grim. I realized how cliché the expression "getting your affairs in order" is because, when it was time to do so, I suddenly had to figure out what exactly that meant. I was sad. I didn't want to die, but things weren't looking good. I felt completely out of control.

That's when I started searching for Ovary Jones. She didn't have a name initially, but, desperate for hope, I needed to figure out how other people blazoned the trails of their cancer journey. Initially, it started in my imagination, as I thought about my grandmother and others who fought before me. What did those brave warriors have in common? What was it like ten or twenty years ago? How has it changed?

Once I was out of the hospital, I started consuming a steady diet of survivor stories. Every day, I learned more about what we had in common, even if the stories I read and listened to were very different from my own. Eventually, in my mind, we were all part of a prestigious club of brave souls that I affectionately dubbed Ovary Jones because it had an edgy, rebellious ring to it. It became a source of power for me that I could tap into when I was discouraged. When I got bad news, I named the emotion I was feeling and then watched a video on miracles or listened to an inspirational podcast. I thought about other Ovary Jones survivors and realized most recoveries aren't a steady incline toward wellness. They involve bumps and bruises along the way. There is value in progress over perfection. Progress means we don't give up. Progress means we keep moving, and it might even mean we get mentally stronger even if, at times, we get physically weaker. Perfection is an illusion and often a stumbling block. Your journey won't be perfect, but you can make progress.

This book is an invitation for you to join our ranks. I've recounted my journey for you, hoping you will find comfort when you need it. These pages are packed with power for you to tap into. *Becoming Ovary Jones* is not intended to be a passive read. There is a section called "Actionable Hope" at the end of each chapter. Action leads to hope. The more you do the "actionables" at the end of each chapter, the more hope you will have and the more mentally tough you will become. Hope is critical in the cancer journey. Give yourself the gift of hope. It takes a little effort, but I promise you, warrior, hope is everything.

Also, at the end of every chapter are "Life-Prolonging Take-aways" I learned throughout my journey. Every patient is unique, and our experiences with cancer are different. You will learn some lessons I didn't, so I invite you to add to the list. What I've learned is that while our journeys are different, there are also a lot of similarities, too. That's why tapping into your community and the Ovary Jones club is so powerful. We weren't meant to travel this road alone. We are better together.

CHAPTER 1

WELCOME TO THE CLUB

Welcome the task that makes you go beyond yourself.

—FRANK MCGEE

Our lives are a reflection of the decisions we make every day. I've said this to my kids from the time they were able to make decisions, and, as a business coach, I say it to my clients a lot, too. I've always been a big believer in the idea that our lives are our fault, and the moment we take 100 percent responsibility for the decisions we make and how they manifest into our reality is the split second when we can change our fate.

Then I heard my doctor's words and saw the scrunched-up expression she had when she spoke a new, profoundly different reality into existence. "You have cancer." Never will I ever unhear that sentence or unsee that look on her face. Obviously my first thought was "No!" I didn't choose cancer! This was certainly not a decision I would ever make. I rejected the notion. Cancer is not my decision, and I was indignant at the thought of it! (Turns out, cancer didn't care one bit whether I welcomed it or not.) Of course, the weeks that followed provided plenty of time for me to grapple with it all.

Nobody chooses cancer. It stinks 100 percent of the time. If you heard those words too, take a deep breath. You didn't decide to get cancer either. We are certainly not alone. Millions heard the same news you did already this year. Approximately 38.4 percent of men and women will be diagnosed with cancer at some point in their lifetime according to the National Cancer Institute. A cure could not come fast enough!

In the beginning of my relationship with cancer, I wasted too many brain cells trying to figure out what I did to deserve such an ugly disease. Maybe you feel like you've been cursed too. I felt like I somehow let my family down. We have enough to process in the early acceptance of a diagnosis—we certainly don't need to add guilt to the mix.

Thankfully, I had people who cared enough to pull me off of my whimper wagon. They helped me divorce myself from the preconceived notions I had about cancer. They helped me focus on finding joy in every day in spite of my circumstances. My mind tried to convince me I couldn't be happy because I was sick. How crazy is that? If we can only be happy in the absence of adversity, our happy time is severely limited! Thankfully, my sphere of influence was saturated with professional business and life coaches that challenged me to shift my perspective and adopt a radically different outlook.

It is surreal to think that my job played such a big role in surviving my cancer battle. After a long career in sales, I partnered with Southwestern Consulting, one of the most trusted sales performance companies in the world. Southwestern Consulting is incredibly successful at transforming people into highly self-disciplined, efficient, and effective leaders through their coaching programs. I am just one of their leadership and business development coaches. When we think of coaches, we usually think sports. Coaches draw out the best from athletes so they can win. Business coaches do the same thing by helping people reach higher levels in their careers in a shorter amount of time. I have been talking about the mental game with clients all day every day for almost five years. Thankfully, the experience gave me a unique perspective and firsthand insight into human nature and how the mind works. I have seen how a subtle shift in mindset can bring goals into reach that had always been evasive. Perhaps even more important than the insights I gained as a coach are the people I met along the way. I am blessed to know all of my fellow coaches, and, thankfully, many of them are like family. They are my circle of influence. I trusted and leaned on them often throughout my cancer journey. They were all on my side, and they lifted me up countless times.

What do a cancer patient, a boxer, and a business executive all have in common? We all face adversity. We are just like you. That's why this book was written. It's about accepting your cancer diagnosis, choosing your fight, and doing it without losing your mind in the process. It's for you. It's about you. There isn't a "good" flavor of cancer, so whatever you've been diagnosed with will be a challenge, but you, of all people, are up for it.

THE ORIGINAL

It had been twenty years since my grandmother passed, and I wished I could ask her how she accepted her diagnosis, where she found her courage, and about a thousand other questions. I thought a lot about that moxie maverick who learned how to drive when she was seventy. Her hearty laugh still makes me smile to this day. She had this spunk matched with an indomitable will that made her an undeniable force.

Of course, many thought her "indomitable will" and "undeniable force" were nothing shy of infuriating stubbornness, but I think my mom has gotten over that by now. (My grandmother lived life with boldness and great resolve, but those around her sometimes watched nervously through the fingers of the hand hiding their face.) My mom was the saint who took my grandma to all of her doctor visits, tests, and treatments. Of course, my dad, brother, and I helped as much as we could, but most of the responsibility and decision-making weighed heavily on my mom as she provided care and dignity to the woman who brought her into the world and taught her how to love. In my mind, my grandmother was an original renegade. She laughed all the way to heaven.

Outcomes are better than ever now, and hope is there if we look for it. I know you don't want cancer, but if you have to have it, there has never been a better time to battle than now. The warriors who fought before you and I were diagnosed provide a spirit for us to tap into as we fumble and feel our way through the uncertainty. I felt alone at first until I realized I had a decision to make. I could opt to angrily reject the bad hand I was dealt and pout (which admittedly were activities I dappled in initially), or I could choose to smile in the darkness. I was inducted into a new club into which my grandmother and all of the other warriors were a part. I was chosen to join the ranks and so were you. I call this exclusive society *Ovary Jones,* a name that has a wiry, pugnacious ring to it because it is chock-full of incredibly brave people with an outlook on life vastly different from the outsiders.

As I started to talk to survivors, I realized I had a lot to learn. Their collective wisdom marvels me. Like you and me, they were plucked from their normal, daily life and sent on a journey that challenged them physically, mentally, and spiritually. I don't know many cancer patients who aren't dramatically different when they meet N.E.D. (No Evidence of Disease) than before their battle began. The experience often shakes their views of life and rearranges many of their once deep-seated beliefs. For most, it's a life quake, but when the dust settles, we can often find twisted beauty and even appreciation for the new lenses from which we see the world.

Of course, in the alpha stages of it all, I was nowhere close to being able to see how any good could ever come from cancer. With the help of the coaches in my life I started to understand and even adopt the special qualities of the "chosen" warriors who fought before me. In other words, like so many of my brave alumni, I was *becoming* Ovary Jones and so can you. I was choosing to adopt a new mindset, the Ovary Jones mindset, that would shape how I viewed my disease and, most importantly, how I responded to it.

HOPE IS ACTION

I think of my grandmother as an original Ovary Jones, but I know there were many who came before her. Far too many unsuspecting souls are inducted into the club every day. I long for the time when cancer is wiped out forever; however, until then we've been chosen to see the world differently and to live each day like the gift that it is.

In the following chapters, I'll share my journey, hoping you will be comforted by the understanding that you are not alone and are inspired to find good in what seems to be dismal circumstances. My prayer is that you find hope, one of the most vital ingredients in recovery, in the actions that you choose. I've heard it said that every cancer journey is different, but I believe we play a big role in how this whole thing plays out. I am reminded often of a quote by Charles R. Swindoll. He said, "Life is 10 percent what happens to you and 90 percent how you react to it."

My doctors kept telling me I was "crushing the mental game" throughout my radiation, surgery, chemotherapy, and all of the relentless complications. You can too! I am not special. My attitude was a learned response, and you can learn it too. It didn't just come naturally to me. I had to work for it just like everybody else. Mental toughness takes practice. A lot of the lessons I learned are a direct reflection of the coaches who were on my side and who challenged my thinking when I needed it.

At a banquet for my son on the evening of my last chemotherapy treatment, I was seated randomly at a table with two other families. Trying to make small talk with the guy next to me, I asked, "What do you do for a living?" He told me he was an oncologist. I laughed and told him how I thought I had escaped "you people" earlier in the day. We talked about my journey, and he too commented on my attitude. He proceeded to tell me how much the doctors believe mindset impacts outcomes. This stunned me. Why didn't anybody tell me this sooner? Dr. Gregory Willis had no idea that our brief conversation inspired me to relive this journey for you.

MINDSET IMPACTS OUTCOMES

That sounds pretty important. I must have repeated those three words over and over hundreds of times in the months after I first heard them. Mindset impacts outcomes. I felt really lucky because that's what I had been working on throughout my treatment, but not because I was told to. It was my focus because developing mental toughness is what my colleagues and I do for a living. I had never thought of applying it to fighting cancer, but when faced with the diagnosis, it just made sense. When I started applying coaching to my cancer, I felt like I stumbled onto something that could actually prolong my life! I couldn't help but wonder, what would have happened if I had chosen a different profession? I never dreamed my job was actually preparing me for the biggest fight of my life. In fact, I was completely focused on helping the people I served and didn't realize how deeply ingrained the mindset principles had become in my own life.

Allow me to reiterate, just to be clear. The Ovary Jones mindset I armored myself with had little to do with me and everything to do with principles practiced all over the world by business professionals, leaders, and athletes. I never thought about their application in healthcare, but it certainly makes sense. I'm not a unicorn. You can develop and practice these principles, too! There are many books written about all of the things I'm about to share with you, and I will happily direct you to some of the books that shaped my frame of reference along the way. I'm not claiming to have stumbled on a cure for cancer nor am I making any regression or remission promises (although I pray every single day that somebody finds a cure). I am saying the mind is powerful. A healthy attitude in the unhealthiest of times is a worthwhile goal. Time is never guaranteed. I simply decided if I only have today, or if I only have five months, or five years, or fifty years to live, I'm going to be happy. You can be happy, too. It's a choice.

YOUR TOP PRIORITY

Personally, I believe that those concepts I learned from my fellow coaches fostered in me a fiery Ovary Jones mentality so much so that I am completely compelled and convicted to relive the experience for your benefit. Even though I was blessed to be familiar with much of the mindset needed through my occupation, I assure you I was still in uncharted waters discovering how to apply it in my unfortunate predicament. While I had (and still have) wonderful family, friends, clients, and colleagues who pray and continue to encourage me, there are still times when we are alone with our own thoughts. I won't lie and say this has been easy for me or that it will be easy for you. I will remind you of how amazing you are, and I'll tell you to hang on because you are stronger than you realize. I will also tell you what my doctors told me. Fighting cancer is your top priority right now. Treat it like the education that it is. It is like getting an advanced degree. It will demand your full attention. It will require study and practice. You can do it!

Of course, your story is unique, but I'll bet there are similarities in our experiences if we look for them. I hope that you'll allow me to join you in your journey. If I can help you, even in the smallest way, to transform your mindset…if I can make just one day a little brighter…if I can show you that you're braver than you think you are…then maybe, just maybe, good can come from bad. Welcome to the club!

Some of the lessons we learn in life have to be taught to us more than once. Cancer taught me some lessons that, quite honestly, I thought I had already discovered. The school of cancer, cloaked in uncertainty, reveals truths you'll learn about yourself in a massive new world full of labs, white coats, and needles. Physicians practice medicine, and we practice life.

At the end of each chapter, I'll share some of the life-prolonging lessons I learned through my journey and some "Actionable Hope" (things you can do to develop the Ovary Jones mindset). I firmly believe that now is a time for action.

There might be moments in your journey when you don't have much energy and you are just clinging to your bed. I've been there. You might think you can't do anything in those moments, but there are things you can do. You can fight cancer without losing your mind. Grab a pen and add your own lessons to these pages as you learn them. This is your journey. It's your fight. Let's do this!

LIFE-PROLONGING TAKEAWAYS

1. Mindset impacts outcomes.
2. You are part of the Ovary Jones club of brave mavericks who came before us.
3. There's no better time than now to be diagnosed with cancer.
4. You can still be happy.
5. Good can come from bad.

ACTIONABLE HOPE

It is time to start assembling a small group of friends and family whom you can lean on when you need encouragement. Cancer survivors tend to have a lot of understanding about the emotions you are sorting through. Carefully choose people who are optimistic and good at listening. These people will be your support team in the months to come. They will play a critical role in your recovery. You are the captain, so be sure to surround yourself with positive people.

What friends or family members do you have who tend to make you feel better when you talk to them?

Who do you know who is a cancer survivor?

CHAPTER 2

THE PREGAME

Sleep, riches, and health to be truly enjoyed must be interrupted.
—JOHANN PAUL FRIEDRICH RICHTER

We had just returned from an incredible mother-daughter week in San Diego, and I was still smiling with the fresh memories I knew would live on forever. My daughter, Kenzie, and I trekked across the country to spend some time with Tabby, her friend from high school, because the new, tough-as-nails Marine stationed at Camp Pendleton was homesick. Tabby spent a lot of time at my house through the years and I love her like my own, so we were all excited to reunite and have some fun together. As an added bonus, a sales manager wanted me to do a workshop in his office to fire up his team so they could finish their year strong. It was a perfect week filled with lots of sunshine, waves, good food, laughs, and just enough work to add a sense of accomplishment to the trip.

Once home, reality slapped the grin off my face pretty quickly. My dad got the diagnosis we all fear. He had an ulcer or something on his lip that wasn't going away, but we didn't think it was going to be cancer, of all things! The following weeks were jammed running my parents to doctor appointments. It was a chaotic whirlwind that climaxed with a massive surgery that left my mom and I clinging to each other for five hours. We held his hands as he woke, and the magnitude of all he was going through rendered both of us speechless. We realized it was going to be a long road toward recovery.

Of course, family and friends all wanted to know what they could do to help. The love and support were comforting; however, truth be told, we really didn't know what to do ourselves. Time slowed down. A friend sent him a card with a picture of a monkey in a tree that said, "Hang in there." (We've all seen that card.) He taped that monkey to the fireplace where he could stare at it throughout his long and uncomfortable days. He had four months before his next surgery and a lot more doctor visits in between, as well as visits from the home nurse.

The driving started to wear on me, and I was struggling to fall asleep at night because as soon as I crawled in bed, I kept getting this tingling sensation in my back. It didn't take but a few nights to realize why depriving someone of sleep is a form of torture. I went to a sports medicine doctor thinking I tweaked something during a workout. She put me on a muscle relaxer, and I skipped home excited for nightfall and a good sleep.

A week later, I returned because I still wasn't sleeping, and, while I put on a smile, I was in a tailspin. She put me on a steroid and again I scurried home excited to sleep. Visiting my parents was challenging because I was trying to encourage my dad without bursting into tears from sheer exhaustion and a sensation in my back that was getting increasingly more painful. While he slowly got better, I quickly got worse.

After much frustration, I decided maybe a chiropractor could help. Several times a week, I'd run to his office for my adjustments and treatments. He ordered an X-ray that looked pretty normal with minor wear and tear considering I was a gymnast years ago. I really wanted the treatments to work, and for a few weeks, I convinced myself it was getting better. Truth be told, I felt worse. Most of my work is done on the phone from eight to five, but I was struggling to sit at my desk for any length of time. I resorted to standing while I worked and convinced myself it was healthier anyway. Eventually, even the chiropractor confessed he didn't know why I wasn't improving.

Back in the sports doctor's office, I crossed my fingers hoping for an MRI. The doctor doubled down and sent me home with an even stronger steroid. She said she initially gave me the lowest dose and sold me on the idea of now trying the highest dose. Once again, I dashed home eager to start the new fix and get some sleep.

Again, I did everything I could to convince myself it was working. I put a smile on my face when I visited my parents and continued to work; however, I dreaded the darkness of the night. Each night I would retire only to be tormented by the tingling back pain. I paced from room to room and up and down the stairs, night after night. Sleep visited only when it was impossible to keep my eyes open any longer.

Usually I love Thanksgiving and Christmas. Buying gifts, decorating, and even cooking are activities I thoroughly enjoy as I sing off key to every jolly jingle on the radio. This year was very different. My dad still couldn't eat, which put a damper on Thanksgiving. I certainly didn't feel like cooking anyway. I had a big leadership summit coming up with a company I had been trying to engage with for two years, so I muddled through the first big holiday and focused on preparing for the early-December conference that I had worked so hard for.

A few days before the big event, my son asked me a question at the dinner table. As I mulled over an answer for him, my eyes wandered up to the ceiling. That's when my thoughts came to an abrupt halt, and I stood up immediately pointing to the vent. "What is that?" The white ceiling in the dining room of the cute little North Carolina townhouse on the lake that I decided to rent for a year to avoid the northern cold climate where we usually lived was in stark contrast from something black growing out of the vent. Immediately, I got online and had a mold tester knocking on the door the very next day. He told me the results would be back in a few days, which coordinated with my return from the summit in Virginia Beach. I would only be gone three days, and I figured then I would focus on this new problem in addition to all the others. For quite some time, I've had a running mantra in my head, "I eat problems for breakfast." It was times like these that I was preparing for.

The night before my departure I crawled in bed begging my back to be calm so I could get some much-needed rest. Shortly after closing my eyes, I felt a sharp piercing on my right temple. I jumped out of bed and ran to the mirror convinced I'd see a spider bite or something. I couldn't see anything, so I convinced myself it was my imagination.

The summit I had looked forward to with such anticipation dragged on. I couldn't sit still because my back hurt so badly and I felt undeniably horrible. To add insult to injury, the right side of my face started hurting and a bright red rash started to appear exactly where I felt the painful piercing a few nights before.

As soon as I got home, I made an appointment with the first

doctor who would see me, who happened to be a resident. I pulled my hair away from my face and showed her the rash that was now on fire, and I told her about my back pain. She did a full exam and mentioned my uterus seemed enlarged but said that wasn't usually anything to worry about. Then she pulled the attending physician in who, with one quick glance, immediately exclaimed, "Shingles!"

Shingles? My head was swimming. Was that the chicken pox thing? I thought I was vaccinated. Maybe that's the one that only strikes people who were vaccinated? I had no idea, but they said fortunately, I caught it early and, fingers-crossed, that meant I wouldn't get hit with the laundry list of symptoms they described. I took the prescriptions they scribbled for me to the pharmacy on my way home, and the next morning, I added a fist full of pills to the problems I eat for breakfast.

By the way, the test results came back...I'd been breathing black mold spores for ten months. I wasn't very happy when I called the owner of the townhouse because I knew there was a problem with the washing machine when I first moved in that caused the water problem, and I also realized she obviously slapped a Band-Aid (in the form of a new washing machine) over a much bigger problem.

Of course, I kept my fingers crossed, hoping I didn't get any more symptoms, but that turned out to be an ineffective plan of action when fighting shingles. By Sunday morning, I was glued to my bed with a high fever and a headache that made me want to curse the sun. I wasn't sure that I had ever felt worse until the phone rang. My landlord, not known for her empathy, called and put me in a three-way conversation with her insurance company. I know they weren't screaming, but it sure sounded like it to me. I tried to tell them how sick I was and how toxic I feared the place to be, which resulted in marching orders. She told me to get out, which I wanted because I had never been chronically sick in my life; however, I had no idea where I was going to go, especially in my condition. We gathered up some essentials and my bag full of pill bottles and headed to a hotel. Surely, we weren't going to be homeless for Christmas.

Fortunately, the flu-like symptoms subsided relatively quickly, and once the rash healed, I could visit my parents. I felt badly that I wasn't able to see them, but I certainly didn't want to risk my dad getting shingles! He had his own healing that he was working through. He still looked like he was miserable, and we were looking forward to January, when he would have his next surgery.

Meanwhile, I kept taking all my pills, but the next problem didn't wait long to present itself. The pains in my back at night morphed into electric-shock sensations that shot through my body like a lightning bolt. I had never felt anything like it! I went to the ER, but I didn't get any answers and was told to make an appointment with a neurologist. The first appointment I could get was in January. Night after night, the shocks intensified. It was the weirdest thing because I didn't feel too awful during the day, but when the sun retired, the nightmares began, except I was wide awake. I used breathing techniques when I felt the shocks surging just to endure them.

MRI, PLEASE!

The whole month of December consisted of trips to the ER, urgent clinic, and a gynecologist because of the comment about the size of my uterus. I told my family, "All I want for Christmas is an MRI." As much as I hated living in a hotel, I wanted to know what was wrong with me even more than I wanted a home. Family is fantastic, and somehow despite it all, we managed to laugh and enjoy the true meaning of Christmas without all the decorations or even the good food. Thanks to online shopping, I even managed to pull off a few gift surprises for my family.

My surprise came a few days later when I got a phone call telling me there was a cancellation and they would do an MRI on New Year's Eve. FINALLY! I breathed through the electric-shock sensations for a couple more nights and sprinted to the appointment. I was sure they were going to find the super pesky bulging disk that showed up for dinner so many months ago and feasted on my sweet dreams ever since.

It wasn't until I got there that I realized I'd never had an MRI, and I didn't know what to expect. They handed me a ball and cleared the room, leaving me all alone with my thoughts. The confined hours passed slowly, but I endured because I focused on the idea that you can't solve problems you don't understand and thankfully keeping still in this creepy tube was going to shine much-needed light on whatever was attacking me each night.

Eventually, I heard life in the room again, and I could breathe a sigh of relief. Ta-da! All done. They told me I'd hear something in a few days and sent me on my way. "A few days," I muttered as I got in my car. I decided New Year's Eve was a great time to say goodbye to the year of uncertainty, and I looked forward to the new year starting with solutions. If "uncertainty" was the one word that summed up the whole year, I wondered what word would capture this next year. Maybe it would be the year I made partner in my firm. Partner. That sounded like a good word. I started to plan how I would make that happen.

As I enjoyed thinking about how I was going to achieve my goals in the new year, my phone rang, snapping me back to reality. It was a doctor asking me to please go to the emergency room. That's when the question I tried not to think about first escaped my lips. "Is it cancer?"

He didn't want to confirm it on the phone but admitted that there was something on the MRI that looked like it. I'm not sure why I expected preferential treatment at the ER on New Year's Eve. I just heard the "C" word! Why do you want me to sit in a waiting room with drunk people who need stitches all night? Nervously, I chatted with the veteran beside me who fortunately wasn't drunk or bleeding. I think he knew my mind needed to be diverted from the heavy darkness that was surely evident on my face. I was happy to let him carry the conversation, and I listened for what seemed like hours, because it was.

Eventually, they called my name, and I stood up to face the truth. It turns out the truth was a different waiting room, a really busy nurse, and more tests they wanted to run. Believe it or not, that whole night ended with no real answers, and a doctor recommending I schedule an appointment with a gynecological oncologist ASAP.

Number 1: I didn't even know gynecological oncologists existed. I immediately realized how naïve I was.

Number 2: Nobody, and I do mean nobody, is open on New Year's Day!

IT'S A BURGH THING

I grew up in the Pittsburgh area, and some of my family was still there. My parents were talking about moving back after my dad's surgery. So, I had a decision to make. One of my coaches told me one time when I was in a crossroads situation, "Don't get stuck trying to make the *right* decision. Sometimes you have to just make a decision and then make that decision right." New Year's Day consisted of soul searching, making a decision, and then packing. I was already homeless, and my insurance company hired a moving company to go in and pack up all my things so that the ceiling could be torn down and repaired. This would leave me homeless for months, and my year in North Carolina was drawing to an end anyway. I called a doctor friend of mine from Pittsburgh and asked for recommendations of the best gynecological oncologist he could find. Once I had a short list, I was ready to make calls as soon as the eternally long New Year's Day was in the history books.

I was up bright and early because I hadn't slept, waiting for everybody to wake up and get to work on the first business day of the year. The first call I made yielded a lot more questions than answers. I learned I needed to get all of the results transferred to Pittsburgh to make this work. Piece of cake! Surely, I could get doctor's offices and my insurance company to work together to make this concert happen, right? If I could, they would see me in Pittsburgh the very next morning. I loaded up my car with as much as I could and started the seven-hour drive, making phone calls the whole way. I was still waiting for the office in Pittsburgh to tell me they got everything they needed while hounding the insurance company to jump through the hoops I needed them to get through. It didn't seem like the challenge that it apparently was. It's a fax machine, people!

Once it was all finally done, I finished the drive in silence. Worry is a waste of time, I thought. Fear is just an emotion, and it's okay to feel it and then let it go. More deep breathing. The drive hurt my back, but, eventually, I was greeted with familiar buildings and then the hugs of people I love.

DON'T PASS GO

Thankfully, my appointment was early in the morning, so I didn't have to practice endless thought-control methods. Dr. Eirwen Miller entered the room like a little ball of energy. She asked me about the troubles I had been having over the previous four months. She had a reassuring confidence even though I thought she looked way too young to be wearing that white coat. It was obvious she was smart, and I had plenty of time to study the walls to see she was qualified. I liked her…at least until she scrunched up her pretty face and confirmed the words the previous doctors didn't want to say. At that moment, I didn't like her too much, but I knew she was just the messenger, and I thought about how often she must have to deliver that awful news. Then she told me she wanted to admit me. "Wait. What? Admit me?"

Now. Do not pass go. Do not collect $200. Whoa. I didn't see that coming! My mind raced as I thought about all of my appointments and my busy, busy life. My schedule is full, and honestly, I like it that way! That's when I first realized I don't have time for cancer! This has to be a mistake! Somebody needs to tell cancer I'm too busy. Cancer is rude.

As I soaked this revelation in, she stressed one more very important piece of advice. She instructed me not to get on the internet. "There's too much misinformation on there, so for your own good, just stick with me for now."

I can't say I've always been known to follow instructions. I actually laughed at the irony because normally I like to figure things out, so I often don't even read instructions until I get stuck. It's my last resort. Now I was told not to read, and it was the first thing I wanted to do. This wasn't a normal time, though, so I figured I'd buck tradition and actually take her advice. Knowledge isn't always power. Perhaps this time, ignorance is bliss. No statistics. No preconceived notions. I stuck to the "no internet research" rule while the cancer was out of control.

Cancer. "Cancer" became the word of the year. It wasn't "part-ner." It was "cancer"...and it started immediately.

Your courting with cancer was probably much different. (I realize most people aren't pushed back into a wheelchair and admitted to a hospital instantly.) Most people have time to process the diagnosis, get second (or multiple) opinions, and participate in treatment decisions.

CHOOSING YOUR TEAM

My chemo sister, Beth Parson, heard the news from her doctor after some tests. She had been having pains and was gaining weight even though she wasn't able to eat much. By the time she heard the actual words, she had pretty much figured it out. The doctor confirmed that it was a tumor on her left ovary.

Figuring out the next steps while sorting through the waves of emotions is challenging. Beth was referred to an oncologist to start planning her course of action, but the doctor lacked empathy and told her she wouldn't make it to see the next year. Discouraged by his demeanor, she looked for another doctor. The second doctor kept referring to the tumor on her right ovary. She knew where the pain was and realized he didn't seem careful with details. Finally, she was referred to the team that was right for her under the care of Dr. Sarah Miller, my favorite cancer wrecker and chemotherapy authority. Dr. Sarah tells patients, "If you keep your face toward the sun, you will not see the shadows." Beth and I met at chemotherapy under Dr. Sarah's care, whom we both adored for her sense of humor and medical brilliance.

Getting second, third, or even fourth opinions is perfectly acceptable. You choose your team. You have to believe they know what they are doing and have your best interest in mind. We have to assemble the best team we can because they play a valuable role in our recovery. When the early doctor told Beth she wouldn't make it, she literally told him, "You can't say that, because you're not God and I'm not claiming that!" In her case, she didn't trust the first doctor, and she allowed her intuition to drive her to seek out other providers until she found a team she believed in.

You have the right to find a doctor you want to work with. You should feel good about your team and optimistic about your treatment. Your recovery will take teamwork. Participate in your recovery actively. This is your fight, and you are up for the challenge.

LIFE-PROLONGING TAKEAWAYS

1. The healthcare professionals are on *your* team…you're the captain, and you pick the team.
2. Take an active role in your recovery.

ACTIONABLE HOPE

It takes a little bit for the news to sink in. I remember not wanting to hear the "C" word, and I wished a whole day would go by that I didn't have to hear it. Truth be told, we can't avoid the truth. Of course, you should get a second opinion. Get as many opinions as you need; however, once the diagnosis is reaffirmed, we need to accept it and then decide what we're going to do about it. Many patients find acceptance through clarity, and getting a better understanding of the facts can be calming. It's all confusing at first. Start to unravel all of the emotions and prepare a list of questions to ask the healthcare team you choose to work with.

Get a notebook. This is going to be your best friend for a while. You can call it your Warrior Notebook or something catchy, but get used to carrying it with you. Write down all your questions. Write down the names of your providers and medications you are on.

What are your concerns?

What are you afraid of?

What questions do you have?

CHAPTER 3

GOOD TIMES
ON UNIT 9

Man never made any material as resilient as the human spirit.

—BERNARD WILLIAMS

The only two occasions I ever spent the night in the hospital were when I delivered my three precious babies. My advice to expecting mothers from then on was always, "If you're going to have twins, have them first." Countless women over the years told me how they dreamed of having twins. Personally, it never even crossed my mind because twins didn't run in either of our families. My doctor laughed and informed me they didn't run in Adam and Eve's family either and now they do run in my family. I failed to see the humor in that as I chased three little ones all over the house just fourteen months apart. Twins, I discovered, are not buy one get one free. As their amazing personalities developed, I realized the only thing they have in common is their birthday. Mackenzie (always called Kenzie) is a chatterbox who knows no strangers. Caleb is more introverted, perhaps because he never got a chance to talk. Caleb is logical and process driven, while his sister is a spontaneous whirlwind of emotions. Their slightly older brother, Nick, led the twins into all kinds of mischievous adventures that I'm still learning about.

For me, my limited hospital experiences were joyous; in fact, they were the best days of my life. I spent most of the first day reminiscing about those two previous hospital stays and how they profoundly and forever changed my life for the better. At the time, the contrast of the hospital stays couldn't be any more opposite, and the thought that this diagnosis could also change my life in any positive way was inconceivable.

This hospital visit was far from joyous and incredibly different from my previous experiences. It was odd because I checked in like it was a hotel. I felt fine during the day, and I wondered what the electrical shocks were going to be like in the hospital. Maybe they would monitor them? I had a lot of questions, but I stuck to my guns and didn't consult any search engines as per the doctor's recommendation, even though I had my laptop by my side the whole time. The night was sleepless but surprisingly shock free. Do the shocks only come when I start to sleep? I had a lot of curiosity.

The scrubs didn't waste any time at all running labs, taking another three-hour MRI, doing a bone marrow biopsy, and getting me lined up for radiation. Honestly, I didn't know if I should be impressed or terrified by their frenzy. I was shuffled from test to test in a wheelchair by a fast-paced transporter who knew all the shortcuts. It seemed as if most of the tests were in the creepy basement of the hospital behind doors that warned of danger and didn't look even remotely inviting.

I was out of my room so much that I almost missed my oldest son, Nick, who had come to visit. He had started writing a note when I rolled in, and I was really happy that I didn't miss him after my long day. Soon the twins joined us, which filled my heart with joy and much-needed optimism. For a little while, I felt "normal" surrounded by my kids, talking and even laughing as we enjoyed each other's company. I didn't want them to see me cry as they said goodbye, so I bit my lip and forced a smile. Then I picked up the notebook to read what Nick had started to write. He penned how he would not have survived me dying a few years ago, but if I really had to go, he wanted to reassure me that he would... his words were interrupted when I returned. He never finished the sentence, and he didn't have to. I understood. I knew how hard this was on my family. When one person has cancer, the whole family has cancer. I realized I needed to talk to the kids about my diagnosis, but the doctors were still doing tests, and they hadn't identified what kind of cancer I was battling. I went to the bathroom and let the tears stream down my cheeks before I washed my face and pulled it together.

After settling in to the not-so-comfortable single bed with side rails that made me feel like a toddler, I called my parents. My dad's surgery was fast approaching, so I wanted to make sure he was ready to get it over with and that he was not worrying about me. As we were enjoying our conversation, a guy started to walk in my room, hesitated, and then turned to walk out. He looked like he was visiting a family member, and I assumed he mistakenly walked in the wrong room. He only took a few steps, and then he turned around and walked back in. I told my parents I'd call them back and gave him my attention. He nervously walked to the end of my bed and introduced himself as my neurosurgeon. It was after 10 p.m., so I was curious why he was working so late and why he didn't look like he was working. He was wearing jeans, a button-down shirt, and a bomber jacket.

The brief conversation was awkward. He asked standard questions about how I was feeling, and then he got a chair and sat down, still at the foot of the hospital bed. He told me he looked at my MRI, and he explained how the tumor was compressing my spinal column. They hoped the radiation would shrink the tumor before it paralyzed me. Then he seemed to struggle with his words, so he blurted out, "I've seen a worse case."

Those words lingered in the air taunting me as he fell silent, and I played a quick game of chess in my mind. To ask or not to ask. Of course, his statement begged the question, "Well what happened with this 'worse case'?" I decided I didn't want to know because he didn't offer any more information. Surely if it were encouraging, he would have continued to tell me about this other patient, right? He stood up and told me he was going out of town for the weekend but that I was in good hands with his residents and he would be updated continuously while he was away.

Every morning thereafter started with residents tickling my feet at 4:30 a.m. and asking if I felt any tingling in my toes or fingers, along with other questions. The radiation started immediately on a Saturday. (I didn't realize Saturday radiation was rare and reserved only for urgent cases.) My life went from a super busy career and endless errands to staring out the window waiting for the next test or procedure. I honestly felt like I was in death's cross hairs. I wanted the doctors to tell me I was going to be okay and soon this would all be behind me. Of course, I understood they couldn't lie to me or give me false hope. After one procedure, I asked my oncologist how long I had, but she dodged the question like a slick politician. Instead she assured me I would have the best quality of life possible and that I'd be comfortable. I insisted I wanted to be here for my grandkids, and she asked when I was expecting them. When I told her there weren't any in the oven, her shoulders dropped. She should never play poker. She admitted I would most likely *not* be around for grandchildren.

Hospitals are a whirlwind of activity, and I was relieved when I finally got back to my room so I could shut the door and start to process my predicament. The evening was full of emotions that flooded through my body and seemed at war with my thoughts. Obviously, I know we don't have tenure in this world, and I felt like I must be staring down the barrel of my fate. My brief future seemed bleak, and I felt completely out of control. As I stared out of my hospital room window on that January evening, the bitter-cold Pittsburgh snow and the blackness of the night matched the darkness in my heart. That's when love strolled through the door. My daughter said she couldn't sleep and asked if she could stay with me. She crawled into the already small bed, and as I held her tight, the paradigm shifted. Life is about decisions.

NEW MINDSET

It was that night, that moment, cuddled up with my twenty-year-old baby girl, that I decided to change my attitude. I chose to flip the defeated narrative in my mind completely. Fueled by my commitment to avoid looking up statistics or any other details of the disease that was attacking me, I chose to believe from that moment on that if one survived, so can I, and if none survived, I'd be the first. That was it. Of course, rarely is a decision like that ever made just once, but for that night, my resolve was strong, and I kissed my daughter as I drifted off to sleep.

Mornings come early in the hospital, and in a flash, my feet were tickled again, vitals taken, blood drawn, and mass-produced food was delivered. Fortunately, I felt pretty good despite breakfast. I felt like a human pin cushion, and the bruising was obnoxious. Dr. Miller came to visit and explained some test results. My "back cancer" started with ovarian cancer. Of course, I had more questions than she had answers, but at least she knew for sure what we were dealing with, and I didn't know enough about different kinds of cancers to know if that was good or bad, but at least one mystery seemed to be solved.

The good news was the radiation was working. They didn't have to tell me the tumor was shrinking. I knew because I didn't feel like I was being electrocuted at night. In fact, I felt so good I started to get bored. Staring out a window all day was driving me crazy, so I walked the halls a lot. My life went from a super-fast pace to a stand-still, and I didn't know what to do with myself all day and night. Streaming movies occupied me for a few days at most.

The news traveled to my friends, family, colleagues, and clients, and deliveries started to flow in. The nurses enjoyed the flowers as much as I did. I also got books, cards, coloring books, and thoughtful calls and texts. The great thing about working with a company famous for mindset performance coaching is the opportunity to meet and develop friendships with the most impressive network of talented people on the planet. Having direct access and being able to reach out to them was huge for me. Of course, coaches have coaches, and mine checked in on me often, which always made me feel better too. I was thankful for the books my circle of influence sent to protect and strengthen my mindset while keeping me focused on gratitude and what I could control. (It seems a little surreal, honestly, that now I'm spending my time writing a book with that same goal in mind for you…to protect and strengthen your mindset focusing on gratitude and what you can control.)

Every day was pretty much the same with radiation, tests, and visits from the kids and family. My daughter, Kenzie, made a habit of slumber parties at the hospital, which lifted my spirits every time. We watched late-night movies, and she even brought snacks. My dad's surgery went well, and my parents planned their move back to Pittsburgh. For the most part, I felt good except my heart rate was often elevated, which the doctors couldn't explain.

Dr. Miller clued me in on the actual diagnosis, which was metastatic ovarian cancer. She proposed a game plan. I would finish the radiation treatments in the hospital, then go home to recover for a few weeks. Then back to my room with a view for a total hysterectomy. After that, chemotherapy. I decided not to ask any questions about staging, and I realized nobody had a crystal ball, so I decided to break this journey down into the milestones proposed to me. One step at a time.

I counted down the days on the dry erase board in my room through the rest of my radiation. They went by ever so slowly. The nurses teased me about never being in my room because I walked the halls of the hospital so much. I found being confined so difficult, and I often wondered how prisoners of war survived for so long in horrible confinement. At least I got three squares a day (satisfaction not guaranteed), new books, and I could walk around whenever I wanted.

At last the day arrived of my final radiation treatment to my thoracic spine. The radiation doc gave me some lotion and warned me about "radiation rash." I was a little itchy but didn't think much of it. I was eager to get back to my room so I could pack and be discharged. (Hurry and wait.) I asked a nurse if some of the flowers could brighten up my neighbors. She was excited to cheer up some other patients with the gorgeous arrangements. That's when I realized the uniqueness of my cancer journey thus far. It dawned on me; most patients aren't hospitalized immediately upon their diagnosis. While I can't say I enjoyed the hotel hospital, I doubt I would have notified everybody right away, so I wouldn't have received all the flowers and encouragement. I also wouldn't have had all the time on my hands to read and solidify in my mind how important it is to search for light in darkness.

Finally, I was sprung. My son picked me up, and, honestly, I wanted to drive as far away from that hospital as possible. I really never wanted to return, although I knew that I had to in just a couple of weeks.

LIFE-PROLONGING TAKEAWAYS

1. Love is powerfully motivating.
2. Cancer happens to the whole family.
3. If one survived, so can you…if none have survived, be the first.
4. Nobody has a crystal ball.
5. Take this journey one step at a time.

ACTIONABLE HOPE

It's okay to cry.

It's okay to scream.

It's okay to be angry.

Write cancer a letter.

When we try to ignore our emotions or pretend we don't have them, we get tripped up. Give yourself permission to feel all that you are feeling. Instead of denying your feelings or trying to force emotional control, lean in and own them.

Admit how you truly feel about your cancer. As if we are on an airplane, we have to put on our oxygen mask first before we can help anyone in our family. That means we need to own our cancer. It's not easy, but it's well worth the effort. Write out your feelings and thoughts. Allow yourself the grace to work through it all as often and as thoroughly as you need to. Write it all in a letter to cancer and don't hold back.

CHAPTER 4

H.O.P.E. (HOLD ON, PAIN ENDS)

Whenever we begin to feel as if we can no longer go on, hope whispers in our ear, to remind us, we are strong.

—ROBERT M. HENSEL

For as slowly as the first half of January dragged, the second half passed with mach speed. My back didn't hurt, and I felt better than I had since I first started my sleepless pacing so many months before. I was hoping to escape the radiation rash, but it certainly caught up to me with a vengeance. Both my chest and back bubbled up and burned. (Hint: if they suggest applying ointment or cream prophylactically, I recommend doing it!)

Free from the lab coats that monopolized my mornings, I

was able to reconnect with the three other coaches in my mastermind group. I'd been having conference calls every Friday morning with amazing women for quite some time. Together we challenge and encourage each other through all the professional and personal wins and setbacks that come our way. For so many months I kept talking about the undefined health issues I was struggling with, and they kept my spirits up the whole time. It was so good to hear their voices and get caught up with their lives. Just being able to focus on somebody else felt so good.

Time flew by as if I were on vacation. My temporary escape from reality ended, and I had to report back to the hospital at an insanely early hour so that we could wait in a jammed waiting room for way too long. I was nervous. Delivering babies was certainly not a joy ride down Santa Monica Boulevard, but at least I got a big reward for my effort. Sometimes pain brings joy, and I got to bring home my angels. I was eager to leave my tumor in the hospital.

I wanted to get it behind me so I could get on with the recovery. My nurse tossed me a hospital gown to change into and got me prepped. My family rallied around bidding me well as I was swept away. I tried to stay strong for my family, but tears welled up and a few started to spill onto my cheeks.

Fear makes the wolf bigger than he is.

—GERMAN PROVERB

I've worked through various fears in my life before, and I've coached a lot of clients to overcome fear as well. A lot of people are crippled by fear, although usually they call it "stress." It's what keeps us up at night riddled with anxiety and why we wake up eating antacids like popcorn. Sometimes fear prevents bright, talented people from achieving their definition of success. Sometimes fear prevents us from doing something stupid and getting hurt. Wisdom helps us tell the difference. Oftentimes the things we fear never come to fruition. I took a deep breath and chose to believe everything would be just fine. Courage is found on the other side of fear. The heated blanket didn't stop my shivering until I decided to pray and put on the cloak of courage. Out I went.

Unbeknownst to me, the surgery took much longer than planned. This was horrible on my poor family. It was only four short months ago that I was sitting on pins and needles in the waiting room anxious about my dad's surgery. I certainly never intended to turn around and put him through the waiting anguish. They hadn't gotten many updates, which invites the imagination to run wild. I know they were worried.

When I opened my eyes, my vision was blurred, and it took a bit to remember what was going on. A perky nurse told me I was doing great, and once the anesthesia wore off a bit more, I would be able to see my family. I felt pretty good thanks to the wonders of modern medicine.

My family was relieved to see me, and I tried to stay awake to visit as long as I could, but I felt like I was suddenly making up for all those months of sleep deprivation. I vaguely remember Dr. Miller telling me she took a grapefruit-sized tumor and a bunch of lymph nodes out of me in addition to a total hysterectomy. For a change, her staff coming in and out as usual all night long didn't bother me at all. Sleep was finally kind to me again.

I will be the first to admit, I'm not a big fan of crazy early mornings. Of course, I've always done what I had to do and often that meant waking up early, but just because I did it didn't mean I liked it. Once I got into my morning routine, I was okay, but peeling the covers back and overcoming inertia was usually a chore. (Isn't it usually that way? We just have to take action, and once we do, our attitude catches up with our body movement.)

Opening my eyes the morning after surgery was a little different. Moving my body was a lot different. I honestly wasn't prepared for how difficult it was, and instead of counting down the days until my release like I did a few weeks before, I was wondering how in the world I'd ever be able to sit up again without a lot of help. I couldn't imagine being discharged.

I found the words of a preacher ringing in my head. I'm quite sure Pastor Joseph Pisano would hope the words he spoke that I remembered in the hospital would have been profound and heavenly. Instead, I remembered him standing at the pulpit one Sunday morning asking, "Do you know what the difference is between a minor and a major surgery?" My mind went to work trying to answer that question, but I didn't actually know how surgeries were categorized. Pastor Joe continued, "It's a minor surgery if it's you going under the knife but it's a major surgery if it's me!" At that moment, I realized I had just had major surgery.

For some unknown reason, to add insult to injury, my heart rate was still elevated. When they woke me up to take my vitals in the middle of the night, my heart rate was 133. I knew from going to the gym and working to get my heart rate that high, something was wrong. I wasn't even disappointed when they told me they were keeping me another night. They ran more tests and tried to figure it out, but they couldn't come up with anything, so they released me the next day.

HOME AGAIN

This was one of the most challenging periods for me. The physical pain was horrible, and I knew I had to heal up quickly because I needed to get ready for chemotherapy. I couldn't even imagine what they were going to put me through next because I could barely sit up. I didn't want to go through anymore, and I knew I had a long way to go. Furthermore, nobody patted me on the back and told me it was going to be all better. I wanted my pat on the back! I wanted a guarantee!

To be honest, I didn't really want to get on the mastermind call with my fellow coaches. It was early in the morning, and I was in pain and cranky. I had to give myself shots every morning and night to prevent blood clots, and I just wanted to feel sorry for myself. I had been doing pretty good avoiding meltdowns since I had adopted my new mindset in the hospital, but as with most positive changes, it wasn't a one-and-done decision. It's one of those things you have to choose every day and sometimes many times every day. At the moment, I just wanted to have a woe-fest. Sometimes when I felt like this before, I would actually set a timer and allow myself a thirty-minute pity party. I gave myself permission to go ahead and let those feelings fly but only for a set time. After that, the worry, the fear, the anger, the resentment, and all of the other feelings I had toward whatever was bothering me had to clear out so that I could allow new guests in. I had always heard two combatting emotions couldn't come to the same party at the same time. In other words, hope can't reside where fear is, so fear has to take a hike. During this particular snapshot in time, hope was losing. I didn't know how to evict my woe-is-me thoughts. Fortunately, it was Friday morning. The power women who have been so influential in my life would wonder where I was if I didn't get on the conference line. I dialed the numbers.

That particular phone call changed my life. Isn't it crazy how we can pinpoint certain moments when we had a course-correcting event that launched us into a new direction? I knew when I opened my mouth that I sounded like a four-year-old and I really didn't care. They didn't mind either because they're true friends; although, I also knew they wouldn't let me go on for too long because they are also coaches. Honestly, I think sometimes you just have to get it out of your system. "I don't want to have cancer," I complained. "I don't want to be a cancer patient. I don't have time for all of these doctor visits. I don't want chemo. I don't want to lose my hair. I DON'T WANT THIS DISEASE."

When I was done with my little diatribe my dear friend, Angie Moss, said, "Yeah, I didn't want cancer either, but you know what? I'm actually thankful I went through that ten years ago."

Wait. What? Angie had cancer? How did I not know this? I suddenly had a lot of questions. It was curiosity mixed with astonishment plus a whole lot of disbelief. Did she just say she was *thankful* she had cancer? That did not compute at all. How have I known her this long and I didn't know she was an Ovary Jones sparkplug? Thankful? Does she know the definition of *gratitude*?

Realizing she rendered me speechless, Angie proceeded to tell us about her diagnosis with breast cancer when she was still contemplating expanding her family. She already had two beautiful daughters and adding a third baby was a big decision. It was a decision cancer ended up making for her. (I had a few choice words for stinking cancer bouncing around in my brain as she relived her story solely for my benefit.) She continued, "Had I not had cancer, I wouldn't have followed the career path I chose and loved and I wouldn't have experienced the success I was blessed with and I wouldn't be here this morning for you." She reiterated that she was thankful for her cancer, and, yes, she seemed to understand (much better than me) what *thankful* meant.

My mind was blown, and all I could do was get off the phone so I could roll that around in my brain about three million times. Thankful for cancer. I couldn't imagine ever saying that with any sincerity at all. As I allowed the idea to marinate in my brain, I started to wonder, what would have to happen for me to be able to say I was thankful for this horrible disease?

Like in the hospital, I decided to have another paradigm shift. I wanted to someday be able to sincerely say I was thankful I had cancer. I needed to choose victory again. I needed to dream. I needed to plan. I needed hope. In sales, there's a phrase "assuming the sale" that means you expect the client is moving forward with you, so you go on to work out the details beyond the initial signing on the bottom line. It was during this time that I discovered the importance of assuming the survival. I figured I could assume victory or I could assume defeat. Assuming defeat kept me in the moment and stuck in fear and wallowing. It wasn't fun at all. Of course, I thought about the possibility of making plans that never happen and wondered if that would be a waste of time. I decided I'd rather be remembered as somebody full of hope and dreams, so I got busy.

Time is all we have. Spending time being hopeful is a whole lot better than wasting time with doom and gloom. I made sure my affairs were in order because I wanted to be responsible. I got all my passwords in one place and documented where I had accounts and all of the things we do to be prepared and responsible. After that, however, I got busy dreaming. I planned, and a lot of what you're reading actually originated in those early days before my first chemo treatment because that was the only way I could ever imagine saying I was thankful for my cancer. If I could give you hope when the moment seems bleak, if I could encourage you to take action and challenge the way you think about your situation the way Angie did for me, then maybe, just maybe, being a member of the Ovary Jones club isn't ALL bad. In other words, I assumed the victory and got on with the business of living. Hope changes everything. Adopting an attitude of gratitude is a worthwhile endeavor.

THE CLIENT WHO CHANGED ME

I had a client several years ago whom I am forever thankful

for because she changed my perspective. Our client's success is always our goal, so on the initial coaching session I always ask, "Why coaching, and why now?" Usually clients tell me they want to increase their income, or they want to reclaim their time because they feel like their business is running them into the ground. Kerry's answer was very different. She said, "My husband of thirty-six years recently passed away, and I know this is going to be a difficult year, and I want somebody on this journey with me who isn't going to feel sorry for me but who will get me focused again."

She got into coaching in September, and she was always in tears when we started each call during the initial sessions. She was such a trooper, and by mid-call the tears would subside, and by the time she got off the calls she had adopted a growth mindset and she always sounded stronger. She hung up with a plan to move forward every time.

The holidays came around very quickly, and I knew she was destined for some dark times, understandably. We had a powerful session about gratitude because in business, as in life, attitude is everything and mindset is critical. When coaches help people frame their outlook steeped in gratitude, it changes their perspective. It is always important not just to talk about things but to do something about the things we talk about. I challenged Kerry to send me twenty-two things she was thankful for in her life. They didn't have to be major things; little things serve the purpose and are often overlooked. The point I was hoping she would see is we can always find things to be thankful for, no matter what.

Kerry sent me an email a few days after our coaching call saying, "Melanie, I can only come up with twelve." As I read her words, I could feel her loss, and I remember letting out an audible sigh. A big part of me just wanted to send back an email telling her it's okay, twelve is good. I certainly didn't want to be too hard on her! We had only been working together for a few months, and I really liked her. I didn't want to upset her or risk her not liking me. I also know I'm a coach and it's not about me. A coach pulls out the very best from people. It was a quandary, but I knew I had to challenge her because that is what she wanted me to do.

My eyes were cringed completely closed as I pressed "Send" on the email comprised of three simple words, "Dig deeper, Kerry." Oh, how I prayed that email would be received with the loving and serving spirit in which it was sent! Just two hours later, I got a reply.

Kerry wrote, "Oh My Gosh! I got home tonight and I realized how thankful I am for sensor lights, so I didn't have to walk into the house in the dark. I let my dogs out and I realized how thankful I am for a fenced-in yard. I got the vacuum out and I realized how thankful I am that I am healthy and I can clean my own house." Kerry continued with more than twenty-two things she was grateful for. I was grateful for Kerry for teaching me the power of gratitude.

There were many times in the hospital and throughout my battle that I struggled to find things to be grateful for. Every single time I got stuck, I thought of that email, and I challenged myself, "Dig deeper, Melanie!"

I am so very grateful that I didn't die instantly in a car accident or something like that. I'm thankful for the "borrowed" time I've been given. I'm thankful that I've had the opportunity to tell the people that mean so much to me how much I love them. I am so very thankful that I can recognize each day as the new gift that it is, and I have learned to find joy even in pain. I'm glad I have friends I can be real with and who tell me little sayings like, "Replace blue thoughts with true thoughts."

My list could go on and on, but initially it was a challenge just like it was for Kerry. Even with cancer, there is much we can be thankful for, but you do have to look for it. Even on the worst day, I challenge you to dig deep and find *something* worthy of your gratitude.

FEELINGS FOLLOW ACTION

Remember how I said I don't really love mornings but once my body is in action my mind catches up and I realize it's not all that bad? I bet there are times when you felt that, too. Maybe it was when you didn't feel like taking that walk but after you got started you realized how much you enjoy (or at least don't mind) the exercise. Taking action is important. Your mind might not be completely on board, but that's okay. If you take action, your mind will catch up.

I'll be the first to admit that there were times that I had no energy at all and even though my doctors encouraged me to walk or do anything I could whenever I could, sometimes that just wasn't possible. There is one action you can always take. You can always find twenty-two things you are thankful for. So that's your challenge. Please take action. Write or record the things you are thankful for each day. They don't have to be big things. Trust me, I get it. There is a lot about this disease that absolutely sucks! I'll bet you can find things to be grateful for, though, even if you can't subscribe to Angie's "Thankful for cancer" belief…yet. To be honest, I'm not quite there yet myself. We're in this thing together.

Mental toughness is actually learned, and to master it, you have to do mental strength training every day. No, I didn't say just the days you feel well. Every day! One thing you can do toward that end is keep a gratitude journal or a jar where you can deposit notecards with your gratitude written on them. During those times when you are really struggling, read some of your entries. (Perhaps you are starting to notice that a fervent theme woven throughout these pages is that your response to this disease is a decision and your responsibility. Own your recovery!)

Another thing you can do is keep on reading, but please be selective of the things you read. We have to protect our mind and proactively choose what we fill it with. There were a lot of people whom I chose not to have lengthy conversations with because I didn't need anybody filling my head with fear. I was working hard not to conjure that up myself, and I had to shield myself from well-meaning people trying to relate but not realizing their stories aren't helpful. I am positive they had good intentions, but I learned to shut those conversations down quickly because my mind was critical to my healing. You'll have to do the same. Your mind is essential to your recovery.

One action my coaches challenged me to take was filling my mind with positive quotes. I've started each chapter with a quote that encouraged me. Have them on index cards taped all over your home. Surround yourself with positivity. Here are some others that spoke to me:

- "Hope is the power of being cheerful in circumstances that we know to be desperate." —G. K. Chesterton
- "I will love the light for it shows me the way, yet I will endure the darkness because it shows me the stars." —Og Mandino
- "Do not let what you cannot do interfere with what you can do." —John Wooden
- "There is no medicine like hope, no incentive so great, and no tonic so powerful as expectation of something tomorrow." —Orison Swett Marden

- "We are born believing. A man bears beliefs as a tree bears apples."—Ralph Waldo Emerson
- "Faith does not eliminate questions. But faith knows where to take them."—Elisabeth Elliot

LIFE-PROLONGING TAKEAWAYS

1. Assume victory. Hope is everything.
2. Mental toughness is learned and requires practice.
3. Gratitude must be our daily focus.
4. Some weirdos are thankful for cancer; I'm determined to be one of them.
5. Feelings follow action.
6. Courage resides on the other side of fear.
7. Your mind is essential to your recovery.

ACTIONABLE HOPE

List twenty-two things you are thankful for.

Keep a gratitude journal or jar.

On days that are more challenging, read some of the things you've been grateful for.

Imagine what could possibly happen that would make you grateful for your cancer journey.

Post positive, inspirational quotes where you can see them every day.

Here are some prompts to kickstart your gratitude thoughts:

Who showed you kindness this week?

Look around you. What things do you keep close by that you are grateful for? (My dear friend and one of my mastermind coaches, Rebecca Swanson, is a very talented artist. She painted me a picture of wild daises, my favorite flowers, when I was sick. It hangs in my room by my bed so I can see it every day. I am thankful for it and the beautiful artist who created it.)

What's the funniest thing that has happened to you thus far in treatment?

If you really *had* to be grateful for something right now, what would it be? Here's a truth bomb: sometimes you aren't going to feel well. Even without cancer, there were times we didn't feel all that great. There were a lot of days when my red blood cells were extremely low and I felt tired and short of breath. Those are the times when we have to go on a mental scavenger hunt looking for things to be thankful for. It's a worthwhile endeavor.

Even the most introverted cancer patients meet a lot of

healthcare professionals. At first, I didn't appreciate them very much, as if it were their fault I had cancer. I guess I was looking for someone or something to blame. Once I accepted my diagnosis, I started to recognize how challenging their jobs must be. I began to really appreciate them for getting in the ring with me. I started thanking them. I'm guessing you have a robust team of scrubs. Who are you most thankful for? Express your gratitude.

Think of a scar you have on your body and appreciate how your body healed. If you are going through chemo and you have a port, think about how thankful you are for that port that enables easier access for you to get your chemo.

CHAPTER 5

MIRROR, MIRROR ON THE WALL

The flower that blooms in adversity is the most rare and beautiful of all.

—MULAN

Angie Moss always has a way of challenging my stinking thinking. She's helped me a lot with judgment. Life is a great teacher, and of course she learns like we all do sometimes. She shared once how she found herself saying, "I'm tired," a lot. She had good reason to be as her life was chock-full, but she realized when she told someone she was tired they would respond with comforting words of pity and reassurance that she had every reason to be tired. She didn't initially realize that the validation she received when she said she was tired became something she craved. It was like a comfortable sweater she put on; however, it wasn't serving her. It wasn't helping her to push past her discomfort. It was her way of wallowing in it, and it was keeping her stuck.

It's like when I said earlier that I'm not a morning person. After years of thinking that, how could I possibly be a morning person? Or how about those nights when you know you have to get up early but you can't fall asleep for whatever reason? You look at the clock and it's 2 a.m. and you think, "Even if I fall asleep right now, I'll only have four hours of sleep and I'm going to be a hot mess tomorrow!" Of course, the next day you have a bad day. What else could possibly happen? You predicted it would be a bad day. We are all susceptible to that kind of head trash. What would happen if we reshaped our thinking? Perhaps we say, "I won't get as much sleep as I usually get, but it will be quality sleep and I will make tomorrow great."

Perhaps you think this whole mindset thing is hokey and not your cup of tea. Maybe you heard of affirmations and you thought that might work for some people, but that's just not you. I accept that; after all, your life is your decision. However, I know you don't need to be reminded that these aren't "normal" times and this cancer thing is kind of a big deal. Different times call for different measures. Let me just encourage you to keep an open mind.

Have you ever paid attention to your internal chatter? You

know, the voice in your head that always seems to have an opinion. How loud does that voice get when you make a mistake? Have you beaten yourself up enough over the years? If we could extract that voice from your head and implant it into a body, I bet you wouldn't want to be friends with it. Usually our mind tends to work against us unless we've worked on our mental game at some point in our life. Perhaps it's a really good time to stop beating yourself up and start feeding your mind some healthy thoughts.

Here are a few truth bombs:

- Your mind is powerful.
- Words matter.
- Preconceived notions are not always true, no matter how often you have (or someone else has) repeated them. Don't believe everything you think!

Even if you've been plagued with a bad case of stinking thinking your whole life, the good news is there is still hope. We can always change. Our outlook frames our outcomes. That's right, it really does impact us *that* much. We can't change the diagnosis, but we certainly can change our response to it.

In the early mastermind sessions after my diagnosis, I said things that revealed my horror and disappointment of my cancer. It's understandable to be disappointed, and the women were more than empathetic. At times, however, they challenged the "judgment" I was giving my disease. By declaring that cancer is *bad*, it closed the door for any good to come from it. We have to be careful with words. If we judge something as *evil*, it will most certainly be so. Don't give cancer that much power.

YOUR ASSISTANT

"Oh, my life is so difficult!" We have something that I think of as our inner assistant that is always on a mission to shield us from noise. We get bombarded every day with a million things, and if we paid attention to all of them, we'd never get anything done. Our inner assistant sorts through it all and only calls our attention to the things she believes we might be interested in. The other job our inner assistant does is super important. She is always out to prove you right. When we have a notion that something is difficult, she will go out of her way to bring us examples of how it is, indeed, difficult. The problem is, she's out to prove you right, even if you're wrong. (It's actually called our *reticular activating system*, but who needs fancy talk?)

The human body and mind are incredible, and the inner assistant has always fascinated me. If you were ever pregnant, suddenly it seemed like everybody you saw in a grocery store was pregnant. You couldn't help noticing all the baby bumps. When you shopped for a car and chose a particular model and color, isn't it amazing how suddenly, as if out of the blue, you started noticing that car in that color everywhere? If ever there was a time to put that incredible mind to work in your favor, sunshine, it's now!

Obviously, I'm not going to say fighting cancer is *easy*; however, I don't like to say it's *hard* either. Those are judgment words. Instead, the ladies in my mastermind group try to use the term *challenging*. That's it. It is not hard, and it is not easy—it is challenging, and you are up for the challenge. If anyone can do it, it's you! If you don't believe me, I beg you to work on your programming and your inner chatterbox.

Maybe you peeked at the statistics. It is challenging not to. Those numbers aren't you. I promise you no matter what flavor of cancer you've been tagged with, *somebody* beat it. You have to believe that *somebody* is you, and you have to believe in your treatment.

There are a lot of great books on mindset and affirmations that I encourage you to read. One of my coaches, Jay Jones, challenged me to carefully write down some statements I wanted to program into my belief system. I repeated them often every day. Pray, meditate, and speak them into your subconscious as much as you possibly can. Jay actually made a recording of me expressing my statements of future truth and put it on a loop that I listened to every night. One thing I used to say all the time that was on that recording was "I have healthy, plump red blood cells coursing through my veins." (I later gained twenty-five pounds during my chemo months, so I dropped the word *plump*, but I laughed at how much it worked!) More on this topic later because it's *that* important.

I don't care how bleak you think your situation is—your reaction is what matters. I've read amazing stories of patients who were given the worst of the worst life expectancy and they're still here! I've also heard stories to the contrary. Preconceived notions matter. Divorce yourself from expectations that aren't serving you. My friends challenged me to focus on things I could control instead of worrying about how many days I might have left.

EXPECTATIONS VS. REALITY

Years ago, I saw a Tony Robbins interview in which he talked about the relationship between expectations and reality. He explained that when our reality doesn't meet our expectations, we're disappointed or often even depressed. It's like we catfish ourselves. Our spirits sink when reality knocks on the door and doesn't look like the profile picture we had envisioned in our mind. Then we get into an argument with reality, but when we have cancer, reality is stubborn. It doesn't cave as easily as we want it to or at least in the time frame that we prefer.

Tony Robbins gave an example of a football player who was

destined to the NFL until a car accident left him paralyzed. He was obviously depressed. Because he couldn't change his reality, he had to shift his expectations to align with his new reality so he could be happy. We have to do the same thing.

I can't change the fact that I was diagnosed with cancer, and neither can you. We can change our expectations about what the future looks like for us no matter how long we are kicking rocks on this planet. Our expectations (the vision we have for our life) can in turn shape our happiness as we forge forward in our new reality.

With the help of the coaches and the inspiration of all the Ovary Jones renegades I met, I decided to own my cancer. It doesn't define me, and it sure doesn't own me; however, I accept this is part of my story. Some say it's the mountain we've been given to move. Find joy every day. Choose to live intentionally. Show up every day even if you can't get out of bed. Be present. As time marched on, I chose to make other lifestyle changes to try to help the doctors out as best as I could.

I had a doctor ask me, "What's it like?" I didn't understand what he meant at first until he said, "Life. What's life like now?" Only one word came to mind. *Intentional.* He smiled slightly, and with just a tinge of envy in his eyes he said, "That's what you all say." I'm sure you would agree that, like me, before you were in the club there were things you took for granted. B.C. time (before cancer) seemed endless. We were going to live forever. Now it's a bit more precious. We notice more.

Everybody's days are limited. We all have an expiration date. We have always known this, but prior to our diagnosis, it didn't sink in the same way. Nonmembers say, "I could get hit by a bus on the way home—nobody ever knows when something could happen." The difference is they don't really believe they will get hit by a bus on their way home, because if they did, they wouldn't go home. The paradigm shift that happens when we are diagnosed is attention grabbing. When you're inducted into the Ovary Jones club by your cancer diagnosis, you join the ranks of people who understand the fragility and brevity of life. Awareness of our mortality is heightened.

It's not all bad when we proactively frame our perspective. Maybe we got a wake-up call and there are things we need to change because, obviously, something we came in contact with was killing us. Maybe we were given some extra time, like an encore. I have no idea, but I'm going to be thankful for it, make some changes to try to prolong it, and live intentionally every single day!

I've heard many stories now about people who were told by a doctor they only had a month to live. Amazingly, as if on cue, they withered away according to the timeline they were given. I've also heard the opposite stories. People like my friend, Beth, who were told they would not live to see the next year who are alive and well. I know I've said it before, but it bears repeating: our minds are incredibly powerful. Nobody has a crystal ball.

As I first stated at the beginning of this book, you didn't choose cancer. What you do get to choose is your response to cancer. Some people choose to fight, and, quite honestly, some choose not to fight. Either decision is perfect if you're making it thoughtfully. It's your life, and it's your decision. If you choose to fight, then roll up your sleeves. It's time to carefully think about your thinking. Take inventory of the thoughts and the things you catch yourself saying repeatedly. Are they serving you? How can you reframe them so that they are building you up instead of tearing you down?

Remember your inner assistant. What you look for, you will find. Have you programmed her to find the positive in every situation? Is she bringing you examples of how helpful people are? Are you finding joy somewhere every day? Here's a challenge: Are you finding something to laugh at every day? (Laughter is so good for us.) Don't shoot the messenger. It was a challenge for me to find humor somedays, too, but it feels so good to laugh. Once we accept the diagnosis and feel good about our treatment plan, it gets a little easier to laugh.

This whole expectations and reality thing hit me hard a few

weeks into my chemo. My first treatment wasn't bad at all actually. I had some new hardware installed (a port), which was weird. I had no idea initially how all that worked and what they meant when they told me they would access my port. What can I say? You learn a lot when you experience new things. A port is a quarter-sized disc implanted just under the skin that connects to a large vein. When they "access your port," they insert a special needle that fits into that port. Then they "hang chemo bags" (which look like IV bags) on a pole, and that drips through the special needle in your port going into your vein. There are a lot of different chemo drugs. I had three different ones that were administered consecutively. Each dripped for a different amount of time. My chemo treatments lasted most of the day but were several weeks apart. Others are treated for shorter periods of time. Some are given more frequently. If you chose to have chemotherapy, your doctors will talk about the chemo cocktail they recommend for you. Each drug is different, and they all have different potential side effects. You don't have to get all of the side effects. You don't have to get any of the side effects. You can work through any side effects as they come up with your team and figure out a course of action that makes sense for your body.

HAIR TODAY, GONE TOMORROW

Somehow, I hoped my hair would defy odds and stick to my head, but that was not my reality. The hairbrush stole more hair every day, and I realized it was getting thin. A friend suggested I reach out to a woman named Bonnie Diver who has a charity in Pittsburgh called "Hair Peace." I didn't know the first thing about wigs. I didn't even know where to buy one. I called Bonnie and she shared her story. She is a breast cancer survivor of fifteen years, and she gave me some practical dietary tips to help me through chemo, like eating miso and brazil nuts. I jotted those tips down, but food wasn't what I was worried about. After sighing, I confided that this whole hair-loss thing was getting to me. I finally just asked her, "What will I do when I lose my hair?"

I will never forget her response. Without skipping a beat, she said, "You'll put on your wig and go meet your friends for lunch just like you do now." How did she know I do that? From that moment on, I vowed to have some wig fun and go to lunch as often as possible. Don't let cancer rob you of any more than it already has. I know my mind will try to play tricks on me and use all kinds of excuses that will further interrupt my life. So will yours. Excuses keep us home. Don't let your world get smaller.

When it comes to cancer, we don't have control over much. As a matter of fact, when it comes to anything in life, there are only a few things we have ultimate control over. We control our attitude, our language (the things we say to others and to ourselves), and our actions. That's pretty much it. Most people spend most of their time whining and lamenting about things they have no control over and very little time focused on things they actually can control. Up until this point, I consciously tried to keep my eye on the bullseye of things I could control as much as possible. It became clear now there was one action I could take to reclaim some control.

I called my son and asked him if I could borrow his hair clippers. I've always had long hair. A lot of women complain that their hair is too curly, too straight, too thin, too thick. I actually always liked my hair. When he showed up with clippers, I put my hair in a ponytail, bit my lip, and cut off the tail. Then I gave myself the *G.I. Jane* buzz cut. The reflection in the mirror was so different than anything I was used to. It actually took my breath away. Cancer had just gotten very real and very personal.

I was disappointed. My reflection (reality) did not match my expectations. I never imagined what it would feel like or look like to be bald. It was weird. It took some getting used to. I had to let go of what I thought I was supposed to look like and accept my new reality. It was a challenge.

Acceptance. It was tough, and I wondered how much more I would have to accept. I thought I owned my cancer, but now I had to accept that the treatment they recommended, and I accepted, changed my appearance dramatically.

It didn't even end there! In one week, I gained seven pounds!

My weight started skyrocketing uncontrollably! How is that even possible? The doctor told me it was the steroid. Within six weeks or so, I gained twenty-five pounds. It was shocking.

Quite honestly, if we really think about it, we have to laugh. I remember thinking how happy I was that while my hair bailed on me and my eyebrows took a hike, my eyelashes were loyal soldiers. I commended them for their resilience! Shortly thereafter I woke up one morning and my eyes were completely naked. I didn't even see them on my pillowcase! They just disappeared like a thief in the night. I laughed. I probably could have cried, but I had to admit, it was pretty funny. My youngest son, Caleb, was away at college, and I couldn't help but imagine how he wouldn't recognize me when he finally came home.

My chemo doctor was also named Dr. Miller. (I joke that they joined forces so it's easier for those with chemo brain to remember their names.) She's Dr. Sarah Miller, though, and I have come to adore her too. Needless to say, I wasn't a fan of the weight gain, my clothes didn't fit, and I needed answers. Her answer was, "You're doing really well."

ROLLING WITH THE PUNCHES

Your journey will likely have peaks and valleys. That emotional roller coaster is challenging. Sometimes the scans and monitoring are a lot to take in. My blood had to be tested every week. My doctors relied heavily on a test that measures the amount of the protein CA 125 (cancer antigen 125) in the blood. For some people, it can be an indicator used to monitor certain cancers throughout treatment. My CA 125 was through the roof when I was initially diagnosed. After the hysterectomy, it dropped by about 50 percent, so for me, CA 125 seemed to be a useful indicator instead of having to always rely on scans. In the few weeks between the surgery and chemotherapy, the tumors started growing aggressively, and another formed in my hip socket. I was sent back to radiation between my chemotherapy treatments. It seemed as if there were much bigger things to worry about than my weight gain and hair loss; however, it was a big ordeal to me. I didn't expect I was going to feel great the whole time, so I could accept the fatigue. I didn't know I wasn't going to recognize myself when I walked past a mirror.

Instead of lamenting the hair that was gone, my support group of coaches and friends encouraged me to let go of what I thought I should look like and be more mindful of my present so I could make decisions for my future. This was challenging. My doctors talked about the possibility of a double mastectomy in my future. I wondered how much more cancer wanted from me. This is probably the time when I was feeling most anxious and overwhelmed. There was a lot of uncertainty. Gratitude actually pulled me through. I kept going with finding things to be thankful for every day, and I found that I could actually interrupt my anxiety with gratitude. It was becoming more of a way of life now. You can do it, too. It takes time. It's a mental mindset shift. It requires daily practice to develop, but I promise it's worth the effort.

The punches rolled in one right after another. After the hip tumor, they told me one kidney was enlarged and I needed to get that figured out. They did a kidney function test to ascertain they were both working in case for some reason one had to be removed. Fortunately, they were both working. Then they ran more tests to try to figure it out.

My heart rate was still soaring, and they wanted me to see a cardiologist. I kept reminding myself how many new friends I was meeting with every new specialist I was referred to, but running to all of the appointments was at least a part-time job. Somehow things seemed to resolve little by little. For whatever reason (they couldn't explain), my kidney went back to normal size, my heart rate came down some, and chemo continued. I was grateful that I was strong enough to get to every appointment. Even my CA 125 came down.

My first lunch date was with my friend, Lori Sadler. I will never forget it because I wasn't used to wearing a wig at all. I felt like I had just robbed a bank and I was in disguise. I tugged at it, worried that it was off center. After a few laughs with Lori, my insecurities faded away. I rocked different wigs and hats for the next nine months.

Celebrate even the smallest wins and victories. If I let my brain replay all of the lowlights of my cancer journey, I think I would still be in bed. Yet another quote I kept handy came from Bill Gates: "Headlines, in a way, are what mislead you because bad news is a headline, and gradual improvement is not."

LIFE-PROLONGING TAKEAWAYS

1. Disappointment comes when expectations don't match reality.
2. You have been given the gift of perspective.
3. Your mind is powerful.
4. Words matter.
5. Don't believe everything you think.
6. What you look for, you will find. Seek out happiness.
7. Lunch with friends is healing.

ACTIONABLE HOPE

Take your notebook to your doctor appointments so you can write down the medications your oncology team prescribes. Use your notebook as a side-effects diary. Write how you feel and anything you're experiencing each day. This will help tremendously as you look for patterns. (For example, I noticed how many days after treatments I needed to keep taking medicine for nausea.)

Use three-ring notebooks to organize receipts and after-care notes.

My team gave me a summary after every appointment, but it quickly became a lot of paper, and it was easier for me just to write down the drugs in my notebook so I could easily track side effects. Many cancer centers have a paperless option and good portals to track your summaries. If you don't go to a clinic with an online portal or if you prefer printouts of your care, keep them in a binder.

Use a separate binder for insurance correspondence. You will start to get a lot of paper from your insurance company.

Keep finding things to be grateful for every day.

CHAPTER 6

THINKING OF THINKING

You become what you think about all day long and those days eventually become your lifetime.

—WAYNE DYER

When people learn you've been diagnosed with cancer, they usually feel for you and want to help. Thankfully, humans tend to be empathetic, which differentiates us from other living creatures. I highly recommend letting positive people in and allowing them to help you.

One of my friends meant well; however, he said something that landed harsher than I'm sure he intended. He said, "It's not like anybody really *fights* cancer. The drugs do the fighting. People just go to the appointments." His comment bounced around in my head like a pea in a tin can for days. I understood what he was saying, but I needed to mull it over for a while.

After much consideration, I realized he couldn't be any further from the truth. He was completely missing the mental battle, which I believe has to be fought first before any healing can take place. Community is important and people mean well, but you do have to be careful and protect yourself from the ignorance of well-meaning friends and family.

My son, Nick, is an amateur boxer. He spends an incredible amount of time in various gyms. When he's not training, he's watching fights. He studied nutrition and meticulously plans every meal to make sure he gets everything into his diet that his body needs for optimal performance. The rest of his spare time is usually reserved for mental conditioning. He knows the first fight he has to win is in his head before he even steps into the ring. Athletes understand the mental game.

The company I work for coaches thousands of salespeople and business leaders every month. They understand performance. The reason why business coaching is so important isn't because people don't know what to do. People often know what they should be doing, but for whatever reason, they just don't do it. We tend to get in our own way. This isn't a unique phenomenon reserved exclusively for salespeople, entrepreneurs, and leaders. Most of us know what we should be doing, but for various reasons, we allow our excuses to stop us. Business leaders, like athletes, understand the mental game.

Patients need to understand the mental game, too. It doesn't mean we have false hope. It means we focus on the things we can control—our thoughts, our talks, and our walks. We focus on the things we think, the things we say, and the things we do. Those are the things that matter because those are the things we can control.

My friend's daughter, a young mother in her late twenties, was recently diagnosed with MS. Obviously it was terrible news, and she had a lot of questions and things to figure out with her doctor. They talked about the pharmacological options for her, and the doctor strongly encouraged a lot of lifestyle changes. Curious, I asked my friend what all they recommended. She said, "They recommended eating healthier, exercising regularly, no smoking, and reducing stress... you know, all the stuff we all should be doing better but we don't." Isn't that the truth?

The million-dollar question is, why? Why don't we do the things we know we should be doing? A big part of it comes down to our habits. Too often, we get so busy being busy that we lose sight of the things that are really important, like exercising and planning healthy meals. By *we* I mean *me*. I am we. Maybe you're different, but that's what usually trips me up. It takes time to learn about healthy habits and a lot of planning to put them into action.

TO CHANGE OR NOT TO CHANGE

Everybody is different, and I am not recommending any particular changes in your diet or lifestyle. That is between you and your oncology team (and nutritionist). I don't endorse any diets or recommend one lifestyle over another. I don't recommend any specific products. I don't even make any judgments about any of the decisions warriors have to make. Some people choose not to fight their cancer at all. Some people choose to keep everything the same during and after their treatment. Some people choose to make some modifications during or after treatment. Others choose to make a lot of changes. I respect every warrior's decision as long as you fully own it. While your team and your family will weigh in on it all, the decisions are ultimately up to you. At the end of the day, it's your life, and it is completely your decision. If we are honest (and now is a perfect time to get honest), I'm going to say we could all improve some of our habits and lifestyles.

According to the medical community, there are either environmental or genetic causes for cancer. Genetic mutations are much less prevalent, accounting for only 5–10 percent of cancer patients according to my doctors. I happen to be in that smaller camp. I inherited some bad genes. BRCA1 and BRCA2 are genes that produce tumor suppressor proteins. Somehow the DNA that makes up my BRCA1 gene became damaged, so it couldn't prevent cells from growing and dividing too rapidly.

This is the same mutation that Angelina Jolie famously confided to the world that she has when she announced her decision to undergo a double mastectomy to reduce her chances of ever developing breast cancer. Her brave declaration brought attention to genetic testing. Had my family been closer, perhaps I would have understood my aunt's breast cancer better and elected to have my DNA tested. (I'm sure that was what Ms. Jolie was hoping for when she went public about her personal health.) Maybe I would have discovered my cancer before it traveled; however, I barely know my aunt. We can't waste time lamenting what we didn't know. Maybe in the not-too-distant future there will be a way to repair genetic mutations. I certainly hope so.

OUR ENVIRONMENT IS KILLING US

The interesting thing is that not everybody with a genetic mutation actually gets cancer, which means something sets it off. Therefore, we're all impacted by environment. In other words, something we breathed, consumed, or absorbed made us sick. There's a famous saying, "Genes load the gun, the environment pulls the trigger."[1] I strongly believe that even though my genes are a loaded gun, I can control my environment better now that I have a better understanding of the world around me. In other words, our genes are not the whole story. Regardless of our hereditary traits, we can choose to see our cancer as a wake-up call and use it as an opportunity to influence the world around us and be careful with what we expose ourselves to.

President Richard Nixon declared war on cancer with bipartisan support in 1971. Unfortunately, cancer didn't resign when Nixon did. Treatments have definitely gotten a lot better than when my grandmother fought, and like I said from the start, there is no better time to have cancer. However, more and more people hear a cancer diagnosis every day.

Of course, it's "not fair," and I have no idea why you and I got sick when other people with the same or worse habits and genetic factors seem perfectly healthy. We've wandered around this planet long enough to know it's just life. Life isn't fair. The sooner we accept that truth, the faster we can get on to figuring out what to do about it. Personally, I chose to make a lot of changes. I always looked at it like I was augmenting what the doctors were doing. I was medicine's little helper. (Eventually I came to believe the opposite: medicine

---

1   I believe the original credit for that saying goes to Liu G. Hannon T in "Reasons for the Prevalence of Childhood Obesity—Genetic Predisposition and Environmental Influences," *Endocrinologist* 15 (2005): 49–55.

was *my* little helper—the bulk of the work started with the mind.) Before we can think about how we can change our personal environment, we have to think about how we think about change.

KICK THE CAN'T

Sometimes people opt out of making a healthy change because they don't believe they can do it. Never underestimate the power of beliefs. Beliefs are at the root of everything we think, say, and do. I know that sounds pretty deep, but let's break that down. Our results come from our actions. That makes perfect sense, right? Action leads to results. When we were in school, if we didn't study (action), we didn't pass (result). That hasn't changed. Results follow action.

How do we know what to do? Our actions stem from our thoughts. That's why we think through our plan of action. We are thinkers. We are planners. We create schedules filled with thought-out activities so that we can accomplish things. That's why I said in the very first paragraph of chapter 1 that our lives reflect the decisions we make. Cancer taught me this is only half of the equation. The second component that shapes our lives dramatically is our response to the events in our life. So, a more complete statement is that our lives are a reflection of the decisions we make and how we respond to events and circumstances that come our way. Either way, our thinking is critical to our success.

Where do thoughts come from? Have you ever thought to yourself, "I don't feel like it," and so you didn't take action? Our feelings direct our thoughts, and sometimes we have to override our feelings and take action anyway to get a desired result. If we only did things that we felt like doing or when we felt like it, we probably wouldn't get much done.

Where do feelings come from? Our feelings bubble up from our beliefs. Those deep-seated beliefs, which we might not even realize we have, sparked a chain reaction that commands our actions, which dictates our results: good, bad, or indifferent. The crazy thing is we formulated our beliefs (intentionally and often unintentionally) a long time ago about most everything. We don't think about those beliefs, and oftentimes we don't even realize we have them. Yet, they are there—somewhere deep inside of us directing how our lives play out. We are held hostage by the invisible beliefs that too often we don't realize we have. If you truly believed singing Karaoke cured cancer, you'd probably be singing from the rooftop.

Think of the COVID-19 pandemic. Governments around the world responded to the information they had about a virus. How each government decided to respond directly or indirectly impacted nearly every person in the world. How we as individuals decided to respond to the decisions government officials made furthermore impacted us. I'm not making any value statements either way about any decisions that were made. What you choose to believe about anything and everything is your responsibility. Our beliefs about how various government officials responded drive our actions during elections. The response to this virus changed the trajectory of many people's lives and businesses. All at once, the whole world got a glimpse into what it's like to get a cancer diagnosis.

You realized you were at a crossroads when your doctor confirmed what you probably suspected. You have deep-seated beliefs about what a cancer diagnosis means that you might need to challenge. We all have feelings of fear and uncertainty that we have to stare down. You will need to practice and develop tools to quiet your thoughts. There are decisions to make and actions to take. This is going to be an interesting chapter in your life.

WHAT DO YOU BELIEVE?

Sometimes we think we don't have any self-limiting beliefs. If you ever wonder if you have a glass ceiling, set a lofty goal and give your brain about three seconds to start feeding your mind with all the excuses about why you can't make that happen. Your mind wants to protect you. Stretching for a lofty goal might make you vulnerable. What if you miss the mark? What if you work hard and fall flat on your face? These are the kinds of beliefs that stifle progress.

Just like a boxer in the ring and an executive climbing the corporate latter, patients have to challenge their beliefs. By far the most important belief I wrestled with was, *can I beat it?* Initially I struggled a lot with that. (Quite honestly, the doctors certainly didn't promise anything but to keep me as comfortable as possible for as long as possible.) Prior to my diagnosis, I was planning on building a house, but I kept hearing this little voice deep down inside telling me I was crazy. It sounded something like this, "Why in the world would you build a house when you might not be around long enough to live in it?" What kind of stinking thinking is that? Deep down inside I believed I was doomed, and thankfully my family, my coaches, and my friends challenged my thinking. That was the biggest change I made. Do you believe you can beat it? I sure hope so.

WHAT ARE YOU EATING?

More belief shifting revolved around my diet. (Again, it's a personal choice, but if you decide to make any changes, work with your doctors and a good nutritionist.) My doctors didn't restrict my diet much at all. "Eat what you're used to eating" was the consensus. The only thing they cautioned me about was deli meat. The rest was fair game. My neighbor, Paul, had prostate cancer. He discovered his cancer early and decided not to treat until he made some lifestyle changes, which seemed to include a plant-based diet. He was getting positive results.

Everybody responds to treatments differently. Some chemotherapy and other medications change the way foods taste. Some therapies, as well as cancer itself, can cause nausea. It's important to get proper and adequate hydration and nutrients to fuel your body as best you can. Some people have a dietitian on their healthcare team. If you have a lot of nausea, the game plan might be finding things you can tolerate so you have nourishment. There are medicines that can help, and taking them before treatment and each day after helps.

Sometimes it is challenging to differentiate between hype and fact because there isn't always conclusive evidence. You and I don't have time to wait for science. We have to fight cancer today, and we have to eat while we are doing it. We have to make decisions about our nutrition before all facts are in. We have to be our own consensus. For this reason, I try to consult multiple sources before forming an opinion, and I challenge you to do the same. While it admittedly seemed like a lot of work because I had to consume a lot of books and digest a lot of information, it was a good outlet for my mind. I felt like I was doing something important. I was taking ownership of my wellness plan.

My son, Nick, challenged my beliefs revolving around nutrition. He wanted to fill his body with clean, healthy food for optimal performance in the ring, so he studied nutrition extensively. He added a lot of healthy vegetables into his diet in exchange for junk food and meat. Taking his cue, I started to study for myself because my recovery and nutrition is ultimately a decision I have to live or die by. As busy as he is, Nick is always up for a conversation about nutrition, which is great. Nick obviously has very different goals, so his nutrition plan is quite different from mine; however, it is great having somebody to talk to about it. If you go to a support group or join the Ovary Jones Facebook fight club, you can find people to exchange recipes with if you decide to modify your diet.

Getting enough and proper nutrition is an important goal. To that end, I decided I wanted a cleaner diet with more vegetables. I've always eaten meat. Some days I ate meat at every meal. I believed I needed meat multiple times a day to get enough protein. I had to learn a lot about nutrition and challenge a lot of the beliefs instilled in me since childhood. The bottom line: I surprised myself. I discovered a whole new world out there full of recipes and a new way of eating. If anybody would have told me prior to my diagnosis that I would go days or even weeks without eating meat, I would have said they were crazy.

There are a ton of "experts" who all have opinions. I read a lot and decided there seems to be healthy benefits when we eat more plants and less processed foods. Several years prior, somebody told me it's best to stay out of the middle of a grocery store. Shop the parameter. For me, this was just the next step. Of course, most food is "processed" before we eat it, but I try to be the one who processes it as much as possible. That means avoiding things that come in cans, bottles, bags, and jars or at least reducing how often I rely on them.

IT LOOKS HEALTHY

In the past few years, the concept of a *health halo effect* has infiltrated consumer awareness. Basically, it refers to how marketing terms shape our beliefs about products. (Again, our beliefs are critical because they influence our feelings, thoughts, and ultimately our buying decisions.) Advertisers are well aware and ten steps ahead of us. They use terms like *all natural*, *low fat*, and *cage-free* to frame our beliefs about the products they are selling us. The images and colors they use on their packaging and displays add to the advertising phraseology on their labeling to create a health halo effect. Certainly, we should all put our best foot forward as we influence the way we are perceived by others. Brands and products are no different.

The problem arises when branding and packaging are misleading. What does *all natural* actually mean? In our mind, phrases like this conjure up a positive connotation, but often that's all it is. Without a definition agreed upon by companies and consumers with regulatory oversight, we are left to guess what these phrases mean. Too often, they don't mean anything at all. We owe it to ourselves to learn about the products we consume. As we do our due diligence, we make our own choices about how we fuel our bodies, and we are less likely to inadvertently delegate our decision-making to tactics used by people in a boardroom trying to sell products.

Take a deep breath. It can be overwhelming. My early thought process revolved around all that I was giving up, and I wondered if this new lifestyle would be sustainable. I went on a quest to find new recipes to try. I ventured into the kitchen feeling as if I had to learn how to cook all over again. It was pretty fun once I realized there was a whole new world of ingredients to try, and I accepted the challenge one day at a time. I felt like I was taking control of something (since my cells seemed out of control) and I was doing my part to help my doctors. As I've said many times, there's no better time to have cancer. Eating a plant-based diet is much more common than ever before, and there are a lot of great recipes and ingredients to explore. If you decide you want to explore some healthier options in your diet, have fun with it.

MATCHA GREEN TEA

Many people rave about the many benefits of matcha green tea. Once I finally started reading about green tea, I learned why. The good news is there are a lot of studies suggesting many favorable benefits. Green tea is a great source for a group of antioxidants known as catechins, and matcha green tea specifically has even more catechins. Studies show that antioxidants like catechins could help protect against chronic conditions such as heart disease, diabetes, and cancer. Because we already have cancer, the question for you and me is, can it help treat cancer? This is another one you might want to read up on. While there isn't anything I've found showing conclusive evidence for fighting cancer, the other benefits might warrant trying it anyway. There are claims that it helps reduce the risk of cardiovascular disease, lowering cholesterol and reducing blood pressure. A study published in the *Annals of Internal Medicine* found that green tea consumption was associated with lower risks of developing diabetes. A study published in the *American Journal of Clinical Nutrition* showed drinking a tea high in catechins for twelve weeks led to significant reductions in fat mass, BMI, body weight, and waist circumference.

Wouldn't it be nice if our bodies would let us figure out one problem at a time? Unfortunately, it doesn't work that way. Just because we are fighting cancer doesn't mean we can't also develop other conditions. For a while it seemed as if I was meeting a new specialist every week because I had so many complications. For that reason, I decided I had nothing to lose with matcha green tea. It has been a work in progress, an acquired taste, but I am leaning in. There is a learning curve as with everything. Perhaps it seems like a lot is being taken away from you, but this is something you get to add if it is new to you, so have fun learning about it. There are different grades of matcha (culinary, which is also further subcategorized, and ceremonial), and it is fascinating to discover the intricate process the tea leaves go through before reaching you. Learn how to store your matcha tea properly as it is very reactive. Some people get a little queasy drinking matcha on an empty stomach, and we certainly don't need anything else causing nausea. Try eating breakfast before you drink your tea. Matcha is high in caffeine, so talk to your doctor, especially if you are caffeine sensitive.

WHAT IS YOUR SKIN ABSORBING?

Next came Kyah Hillis, a friend who challenged my thinking yet again. I was completely focused on breaking up with overly processed foods and changing lifelong culinary habits, but somehow, I missed thinking about the largest organ of our body—our skin. Kyah was telling me about the skin-care products she gave up so she could avoid the absorption of potentially harmful toxins. She started making more informed choices about the ingredients in the products she uses. It made perfect sense and she has gorgeous skin, so obviously she was doing something right.

I started trying to read all the labels on my makeup, soaps, cleaning products, and anything else I came in contact with. I was blown away by all the complicated ingredients. Changing the products I put on my skin seemed like a much easier change than my diet until I realized how many products we come in contact with every day.

Once I started researching, I learned there has been a whole movement brewing of people like Kyah wanting more user- and environment-friendly products. Maybe you got the memo long before I did. I really felt like I must have been living under a rock. Some women have been "girl-cotting" some toxin-laced products for years! As with everything, there are two sides to every story. There isn't conclusive evidence. We have to make some decisions before all of the facts are in, but it's our responsibility to do just that.

TOXIC EXPOSURE

I knew about asbestos and lead paint. I had heard about pesticides and a few other potentially hazardous chemicals used around the house. I even heard about the dangers of BPA in plastic. I had no idea until I started reading that some laundry detergents contain formaldehyde. (Isn't that the stinky stuff that the frogs we dissected in high school biology came in?) I discovered other controversial ingredients. Then I started reading about deodorant! Oh my! I wondered why some of these ingredients aren't prohibited. It's complicated.

As with nutrition, this is another subject of controversy that requires some homework and decisions made today prior to facts that could surface in the future. (We all thought that baby powder was safe, and we sprinkled that stuff everywhere.) I think it's important to read both sides of an argument and then be your own judge. We don't have time for lobby-influenced, double-blind, placebo-controlled studies yielding conclusive evidence agreed upon by everybody. We have cancer *now*. We have to figure out what we are comfortable with based on the information we have today. We have to decide what we rub into our skin that gets absorbed into our bodies.

READ THE INGREDIENTS LIST

If you can pronounce the ingredients in the products you use every day, you're doing better than me. What are all of these things for? How am I supposed to make an informed decision when I'm not a dermatologist and I barely passed chemistry? Initially I thought perhaps I should head into the kitchen and make my own skincare products. Surely Pinterest has all kinds of great concoctions. I've been making my own vegetable stock, so why not? I was thinking preservatives found in skincare products must be bad, right? Then I thought about what preservatives do. They help keep mold out, and I instantly had flashbacks of the mold exposure in the beginning of my cancer journey. I shuttered to think about bacteria getting into my skincare routine. Personally, I decided I should probably leave the chemistry to the chemists; however, that doesn't mean I can't understand ingredients better.

When you start to dig into it, you're going to find there is a lot of hype and some facts, and you will need to decipher between the two. At the end of the day, you have to choose products that do what they are supposed to do without doing harm or causing allergic reactions or irritation. Marketers have one job, and that is to garner interest in their products. To that end, they are usually not above throwing a little mud on their competition even if they know their claims are false. Certain ingredients are demonized—sometimes for valid reasons and sometimes it's hype. Regardless, health halo effects are created in skincare just as they are in the food industry. What does *all natural* anything actually mean? What do claims like *dermatologist tested, clean,* and *hypoallergenic* actually mean? Nothing. At least, there are no regulations in the industry, so there are no agreed-upon definitions for these terms. They are usually used as marketing ploys to make you believe their product is worth more of your hard-earned dollars. Ignorance used to be bliss, but now we have cancer. We can't let marketers influence our decisions.

PARABENS

There is a lot of fuss about parabens. I had never even heard of them, and I was surprised to see such a controversy over a subject I knew nothing about. One of the first things I learned was they are banned in Europe. All of the regulatory societies in the United States have continued to deem them perfectly safe. Apparently, Europe decided to come down on the side of caution and ban them because they think they lack safety data. Parabens play an important role in deodorants, moisturizers, and makeup, providing biocides to the products. They protect the products from contamination, so we are not smearing bacteria, yeast, or mold on our faces, which was my concern with DIY products. There was a study from 2004 that showed parabens present in cancerous breast tissue; however, it didn't show how many parabens were present in normal breast tissue. Many in the medical community say that just because something is present in cancerous tissue doesn't mean it is the cause of the disease. There are also studies that show parabens in a petri dish and in mice have estrogen-like effects; however, humans metabolize parabens much differently and quickly into something that does not have an estrogen-like effect at all. Science does seem to show parabens are rarely irritating and the least sensitizing while doing their job most effectively. While I worry about DIY skincare, I have no problem with DIY reading. After doing your homework, if you decide to break up with parabens, there are many products out there that use alternative preservatives.

FORMALDEHYDE

It is actually impossible to escape formaldehyde exposure completely because it is released into the environment from refineries and it is in so many products that we come in contact with every day. It also occurs naturally so it is not just a chemical product. It is produced in our fireplaces and by our cars idling. It is also a combustion byproduct of tobacco smoke and fuel-burning appliances, along with artificially scented candles. It is found in resins used in pressed wood and flooring, carpeting, upholstery, insulations, and other household products. It can also be found in eye creams, nail polishes, shampoos, and a lot of other skincare products. It can also be found in pet-care products. It is a *known* human carcinogen (upgraded from probable), and prolonged exposure can cause various types of cancers, respiratory issues, headaches, and chronic fatigue. It can contribute to joint pain and other ailments. Formaldehyde can accumulate in the body over time. Products containing formaldehyde do not list it in their ingredients list as such. It is instead listed by a long list of hard-to-pronounce pseudo-names. My best recommendation for avoiding formaldehyde as much as possible is to look for household cleaning products, laundry detergents, and skincare products that are actually labeled "formaldehyde free."

FRAGRANCES

Natural and synthetic fragrances are common ingredients in skincare products. They are often lumped together and listed as fragrance, perfume (perfum or aroma), linalool, or limonene. Fragrances commonly cause sensitizing. If you don't immediately react to fragrances, you might think you can tolerate them and they aren't harmful for you. Unfortunately, though, you might not see the damage on the skin's surface; they could be silently damaging your skin every day. Even natural essential oils and fragrant ingredients can be destructive under the surface of the skin. There are a lot of companies that are proud of their ingredients lists and are quick to highlight the fact that they are formulated fragrance-free.

There is a whole world of products that are gentler for your skin and the environment. I've been having a lot of fun trying new products in my home and on my skin, leading me to say, once again, there's no better time than now to have cancer.

Here's some good news. Since grade school, I have been a dermatological nightmare. I often had red rashes on my elbows and knees, and my mom used to drag me out of school every week for a shot from the doctor. The crazy thing is that doctor died, and to this day, nobody knows what exactly he was injecting me with for all those years. Thankfully, I somehow grew out of most of the eczema on my body, but my scalp remained problematic. I can't even remember how many dermatologists I've been to over the years. I wondered what my scalp would be like when I lost my hair. Interestingly, I had no issues at all. Then my hair started to grow back, and I got my shampoo and conditioner out, excited that I finally had something to wash again. Instantly my scalp rebelled with dryness and flakes. My hair wasn't long enough to hide it, and I was shocked how quickly it happened. How could my head be allergic to hair? Over the years I tried everything from prescription-strength shampoos to ointments, as well as every brand I could find in the stores, searching for something that worked. Because my hair was so short, I still could use a bar of soap, and when I returned to washing my hair that way, the dryness cleared up as quickly as it appeared. When I had long hair, it was hard to see how products reacted with my scalp. This was an opportunity to see almost instantly what products irritated my skin, so I tried a lot of them. I stumbled on a product formulated without sodium lauryl sulfate (SLS), parabens, artificial colorants, formaldehyde, metallic aluminum, triclosan, or toluene. It is the only product in my lifetime that hasn't caused instant dryness and flaking. The only thing I can figure is I am highly sensitive to one of those things that is a staple ingredient to all of the formulations sold when I was growing up. While it's not 100 percent cured, I would say it's 90 percent better, which is a huge improvement for a lifelong problem.

DRY SKIN AND SUN EXPOSURE DURING TREATMENT

Consult with a dermatologist and your oncologist, especially if you have any specific problems like sores or rashes. Skin reactions are common during various cancer therapies. Most traditional chemotherapy drugs are a form of cytotoxic therapy (*cyto* refers to cells, and *toxic* means poison). These drugs are employed to kill cancer cells. The downside is that they cannot distinguish between cancerous cells and healthy cells.

So, they kill them all. Targeted therapies disrupt the activity of specific molecules that promote the growth of cancer cells. Immunotherapy stimulates the body's immune system to fight cancer. All of these therapies and radiation can cause changes to the skin. Some people experience redness, dryness, and peeling. Some might experience autoimmune skin eruptions.

Dry skin (xerosis) can be uncomfortable, and to add insult to injury, we tend to wash our hands more frequently because we know our immune system is compromised. To try to stay ahead of the game, moisturize immediately after you dry your hands every single time. Typically, ointments are superior to creams and lotions at providing moisture, which is why if you have a rash or broken skin, your doctor will likely recommend using an ointment until it heals. Ointments are 80 percent oil and 20 percent water. A simple petroleum jelly without added ingredients was most helpful for my radiation rash. The preservatives and especially fragrances in other products might have further irritated my problem. Creams are good when your skin is dry, but you don't have an actual rash. They are 50 percent oil and 50 percent water. They tend to moisturize more than lotions, which have a higher percentage of water.

Also, important especially during treatment is sun protection and sunscreens. Many therapies and antibiotics increase susceptibility to sunburns (UV radiation) even through a car windshield or on cloudy days when the sun doesn't seem intense. This can be a catch-22. It's important to protect our skin from overexposure; however, we don't want to quarantine for a year and miss the benefits of sunlight and the quality of life we get when we are out spending time with family and friends. Fortunately, we can be diligent and use sunscreen every day. A lot of makeup has sunscreen in it, and there are even sunscreen touch-up powders (not just for women) that you can carry with you for ease of use on your face throughout the day.

EXERCISE

Early on, I know how hard it is even to think about exercise. My doctors told me that, as crazy as it sounded, the only thing to combat fatigue is the very last thing patients want to hear...exercise. They told me even just a little walking will do the body good. It was a challenge. There were days I would get up and walk the ten steps or so into my bathroom, take a shower, and just the standing and that little bit of walking led me straight back to bed for a nap. Listen to your body. Rest when you need to and nap when your body tells you to.

One of the fears I hear a lot about is whether or not your energy levels will ever return. Will this be my new normal? I worried about that, too. It sure did seem like it. I had a scar straight up my abdomen, I had to lift my leg in and out of my car because of reduced mobility from the tumor in my hip, and I felt like I was 139 years old. If you are patient and if you just try to move your body, it gets better.

LIFE-PROLONGING TAKEAWAYS

1. The mental game has to be fought first before healing can take place.
2. Protect yourself from the ignorance of well-meaning people.
3. Beliefs are powerful.
4. Programming is your responsibility.
5. Change is a decision.
6. We live in a toxic world.
7. Exercise reduces fatigue.

ACTIONABLE HOPE

What beliefs do you have about your recovery?

Create your own wellness plan including any nutrition and lifestyle goals.

Think about your lifestyle. Are there any changes you can make that could help your doctors and assist in your long-term recovery?

On a scale of 1 to 10, how would you rate your diet?

What products are you coming in contact with every day that might be making you sick?

Are you moving your body enough?

How can you incorporate more walking into your daily routine?

What time of the day can you make that happen?

When will you start?

Try some green tea.

CHAPTER 7

HABITUALLY YOURS

In any given moment we have two options: to step forward into growth or step back into safety.

—ABRAHAM MASLOW

Taking an active role in our recovery is empowering. There are a lot of ups and downs and twists and turns throughout the cancer journey. We cannot control how our body responds to various treatments and drugs. We have to keep our minds nimble and adapt to changes while continuing to challenge our beliefs and maintaining focus on the things we can control. Once you've spent some time thinking about your wellness plan, it will feel good to try to adopt some new, healthy habits.

In the days and years before your diagnosis, you might not have had much interest in trying new things. Maybe you have some habits you know aren't healthy that you've tried and failed to kick. What I know for certain is there's no better time than the present to actually succeed in lifestyle changes. For many, a cancer diagnosis is very motivating. I know people who had smoked cigarettes for decades who successfully quit for good. I know people who had never exercised who now have movement built into their daily routines. I know people who drastically changed their diets. Many people decide to see their cancer as the wake-up call they needed and an opportunity to make dramatic lifestyle changes in areas they were never successful at changing before. For many, cancer is quite motivating. Apparently, our lifestyle was not impervious to cancer, so perhaps we can adopt some habits that will help the doctors out.

CREATING STICKY HABITS

Unfortunately, our subconscious, where our beliefs reside, is stubborn. It would be nice if when we realized we need to make an alteration to our beliefs, which gets played out through our habits, we could just holler down and give our subconscious the change in plan. It doesn't work that way. Our subs are stubborn. It takes a lot of conscious repetition and reprogramming to replace our beliefs and create habits that stick.

If we need the strength to fight cancer, we'd better believe we are strong! We need to believe we are resilient, odds-defying, and that we have the moxie to get through anything. That's the Ovary Jones mindset. Chances are you might not have those beliefs completely dialed in. I sure didn't. However, you can't let that stop you, and neither could I. It is 100 percent your responsibility to proactively ingrain in your mind the beliefs that manifest into your actions and create your habits, which play out through your actions.

In many ways I felt like I was back at the very beginning of my career just after college. I was hired at McGraw-Hill Publishing Company as a copywriter. Eager to make my mark and prove myself, I accepted my first assignment. My manager pointed to a wall lined with file cabinets all packed with thousands of adverts for books. She handed me a manuscript that was about to be published and instructed me to go through those drawers for inspiration and write the ad prep copy in a similar fashion to all those written before and shoved into files. I worked very hard and was quite proud of the creative piece I submitted. In fact, I couldn't wait for the praise that was coming my way. Face down on my desk the next morning was my first professional assignment. With a big smile on my face, I flipped it over eager to read all the nice comments like those written by my professors in college. To my dismay the only feedback I got was "Start with a blank page" written in big red letters. Disappointment was an understatement. That's exactly how I felt about some of the lifelong beliefs I held so dear. How in the world was I going to divorce myself from things so deeply ingrained and start with a blank page? I had to consciously think about everything I did and start from scratch, learning to change my habits.

TAKE BACK YOUR POWER

Chaos is a natural state. We don't have to try for messy. Clutter comes naturally. We have to constantly work on keeping things tidy. Our minds are no different. When left in neutral, our minds tend to drift into a messy, negative state. A defeatist attitude is easy. It's our default setting. We have to work on our thought life to protect our minds and steer them away from the natural disheveled state. If you are going to win the mental game in this battle, chances are you are going to need to develop some tools to help you clean up your thoughts. Instead of leaving your mind in neutral, you have to focus it. These tools all take practice. They take time. They aren't natural. You have to work for it; however, the payoff is the best gift you could give yourself. These tools rob cancer of the power you gave it when you were diagnosed and give that power back to you. The three tools I learned to use the most in my cancer journey are affirmations, prayer, and meditation.

AFFIRMATIONS

Perhaps we're getting into a subject you once rolled your eyes at, or maybe you have some experience with affirmations. Personally, early in my career I used to think they were too far out there for me and my logical brain. As previously mentioned, with the help of my coach, Jay Jones, I discovered the power of the mind and how to focus it. He taught me how to write affirmations in the present tense, and he carefully reviewed each one I wrote to ensure it was worded in the best positive way so I was affirming what I really wanted in my toolbox of healing beliefs. Words are powerful.

When I had to memorize something in school, I had to take out a piece of paper and write it over and over until my hand hurt. Then I would close my eyes and try to recite it. If I couldn't, I wrote it some more. Finally, it would stick. That's how I learned. That's how affirmations work. You can't say them once and expect them to take root. You've got to drill them down, but eventually they do take hold.

There have been presidents, CEOs of major companies, and people of all walks of life who used affirmations to program their beliefs so they could change their habits. I mentioned earlier how I used an affirmation about my plump, healthy red blood cells coursing through my veins. I said it so often, I truly believed my body was getting better. I used a lot of affirmations throughout my career, so it only made sense that I use this tool in my healing too.

You can write your own affirmations specific to the challenges you personally face. You can build up any area of your life with affirmations. There are entire books dedicated to the practice of affirmations and how to write them effectively. Here are just a few more powerful statements you can drill into your mind through repetition:

- I have today, and today I am a survivor.
- My wellness plan is working.
- I find joy in every day.
- I choose thoughts that empower me.
- I feed my mind by dwelling on positive, constructive, and healing thoughts.
- I am able to relax. I am calm.
- Challenges are gifts. This is an opportunity to learn.
- I have strength, power, and confidence.
- My mind dwells only in thoughts that create health, harmony, balance, and well-being within me and in the world around me.

PRAYER

Be still and know that I am God.

—PSALM 46:10

We have free will. We can choose to believe or not believe in a higher power. That is entirely up to you. If you choose to believe, there are plenty of deities and religions to choose from and then lots more choices drilling down into the details. The decision is yours, and as the saying goes, the failure to make a decision is a decision.

In his book *12 Keys to a Healthier Cancer Patient*, Patrick Quillin writes, "There has long been a link between faith, religion, and health. Studies have found that attending regular spiritual services may reduce mortality by 55%. If worship were a patentable drug, it would be a blockbuster."

To me that sounded like a pretty compelling reason to at least be open-minded even if that door has always been closed and locked. In fact, faith seems to be a reoccurring topic of discussion among cancer patients, even if it is a bit less politically correct to talk about mainstream. Apparently, when we have a life quake, we think more about the end game.

Have you thought about your life's purpose? What's the point of it all? Were you put here just to go through the motions? Were you created, or did you just happen? C. S. Lewis said, "Human history is the long terrible story of man trying to find something other than God which will make him happy."

Personally, I choose to believe in Jesus Christ as my Lord and Savior. In my mind, my faith isn't perfect, but thankfully, He is. I believe we will all have to answer someday for our beliefs. My oldest son challenges me sometimes by asking me, what if I'm wrong? How can you believe in something you can't see or touch? How can you be so sure of something that happened before you were born somewhere in a place you've never been?

Well, I couldn't see or touch my cancer, but it sure did let me know it was there, just as the Holy Spirit does. My question back to my son is always, "What if I'm right?" If I'm right, then the grace of God has been extended to me simply by faith that the action of Jesus Christ dying on a cross paid a price I owed (because let's face it, I've sinned, and so have you). He was the only one who could take away my sin debt. He did it for love. He died. I'm forgiven. That means my citizenship is in Heaven, and cancer or any other disease or mishap will not be the end of my story. That sounds like a pretty good deal to me.

That's only scratching the surface, though. The peace of mind and clarity I discovered in the early stages of my battle were incredible. Let's face it. We don't sit around thinking about our own mortality much. Even as a Christian, I rarely thought about the end. That sure did change when they dropped the evil "C" word on me! I wrestled with it a lot at first. Many cancer patients do.

Prayer always confused me. In fact, just before the pain in my back started, I confided in Preacher Perry Lemmons of Royal Grace Bible Church that I didn't really under-stand the point of prayer. It went something like this: "God knows everything, right? Then why does He want me to tell Him about things He already knows?" The preacher smiled, understanding I had it backward. I thought prayer was for God. I discovered prayer was for my benefit and learning, not for informing God of something He didn't know. Getting silent and alone with God in my thoughts gives Him space to provide the clarity I seek.

God isn't a genie in the sky waiting to grant us all of our wishes. If that were the case, nobody would ever die, we would all be wealthy, and cake wouldn't have calories. Prayer helps us discover lessons in our trials and tribulations, and it helps us grow in our faith. My cancer journey helped me understand the power of prayer better than any other period in my life. In my darkness, I found solace. My fears subsided as I looked to my Father in prayer.

I'm thankful I learned to read the Bible and the grace program that has been freely offered to you and me. Prayer and my faith got me through many challenging times, and I'm sure they will get me through more to come. I wish this world wasn't full of cancer, evil, and troubles, but it is, and I am sure looking forward to an eternity free from heartache and pain. Cancer renewed and deepened my faith. We always wonder how we would react if we were in different situations or experiencing unique traumas. It's all speculation. For me, I learned that I will fight with everything I have to stick around, but I have a deeply satisfying peace knowing I am ready and willing to go home when called. To me, faith is a win-win. The choice is yours.

MEDITATION

Thoughts become perception, perception becomes reality. Alter your thoughts, alter your reality.

—WILLIAM JAMES

Cancer is stressful. Trying to keep calm and lie flat in an MRI machine or during radiation is challenging. Wondering what's going to happen next is unsettling. Living with pain is challenging. Opening the bills and wondering about the financial devastation is alarming. Even before we were diagnosed, I'm guessing we all had an unhealthy relationship with stress. Let's face it, being alive is stressful, and too many of us live with daily, chronic stress.

Our bodies are not built to handle a lifestyle of chronic stress. Stress serves a purpose. We rely on acute positive stress to release chemicals into our bodies that help us perform better so we can accomplish things. Problems arise when stress becomes a lifestyle.

Our body's response to stress is controlled by the autonomic side of our nervous system. This is the side where things happen without us having to think about it. It's all involuntary. There are two branches in the autonomic nervous system: sympathetic and parasympathetic. The sympathetic branch (fight or flight) reacts to stress by releasing chemicals like cortisol and adrenaline, which increase your heart rate and blood pressure and push more blood flow to your brain, muscles, and heart so you can think fast and run fast. Then when the stress is over, the sympathetic branch (rest and digest) enables you to recover from the burst of activity.

Chronic stress creates problems. Continued exposure to cortisol and the hormones that regulate stress interrupts the activation of our relaxation response. If your body is always in emergency response, attention is diverted away from really important activities like building up your immune system. Chronic stress makes us vulnerable. It can lead to high blood pressure and cardiovascular disease and a whole lot of other problems. When you learn to meditate, you discover how to calm your emotions and liberate your mind.

Meditation is an opportunity to hit the reset button. It's like taking a much-needed, well-deserved break. It is the art of being present in the moment, fully accepting the here and now. You might have thoughts in the back of your mind, but you notice they start to settle. Your mind might be crowded and cluttered. Meditation helps you create space so you can embrace calmness and peace. Perhaps you have always been too busy to fuss with sitting still. Again, cancer can be a great motivator, providing an opportunity to learn the art of meditation.

When getting started, one of the easiest things to learn to focus on is your breath. Usually we don't think about our breathing. It is another function controlled by the autonomic nervous system. As you learn to meditate, you learn to quiet and shift out of "fight" mode and trigger the relaxation response. Instead of allowing your breathing to be involuntary, focus on it. Observe it. Take control of it.

There are many books and apps you can tap into as you learn. Some recommend various counts to regulate the length of time you inhale, hold your breath, and exhale. For example, inhale for the count of four and exhale for the count of five. Some challenge you to imagine your breath entering your body as a color like red and see it flowing through your lungs and out into your body, eventually exhaling as a different color like blue. Another form of meditation is using a mantra and focusing on just one syllable. The idea is to calm the stressed mind cluttered with conflicting thoughts. It helps you clean up the mental shop through the power of focusing on just one thing.

I was one of those never-very-good-at-sitting-still types. From sunrise to sundown my body was always in motion because I was always on the go. I never wanted to slow down. I've said it before: I didn't have time for cancer, but cancer wasn't going to wait and make an appointment. I was admittedly pretty bad at meditation at first, but it was something I could try to do even on the worst days when I couldn't accomplish much.

I had a very low red blood cell count for an entire year. I struggled with extreme fatigue a lot. I used to imagine oxygen entering my body, and my blood cells distributing it to all of the muscles all the way down to my toes. I felt calmer with every deep breath I took. As I practiced, my out-of-control thoughts started to fade away as I pictured my little red tanks carrying oxygen.

Several years ago, one of my colleagues told me about a "silent retreat" he went to for several days. (Think monk-like environment, sitting on the ground in complete silence as time drags for a whole weekend.) Nobody talks? They charge money for this? Inconceivable! To me, it sounded like torture, but he said he certainly noticed details about himself he had never known.

I've now spent many hours of my life in MRI tubes, CT scans, and holding my breath for radiation and imaging. Learning to meditate has helped me tremendously with these procedures. I am a work in progress, but meditation has been around for generations helping people lower their blood pressure, ease stress, reduce pain, fight addictions, control anxiety, improve sleep, and much more. Learning to quiet the mind has lots of benefits. It takes practice, but you'll get better at it and it will help tremendously when anxiety knocks.

LIFE-PROLONGING TAKEAWAYS

1. A cancer diagnosis can be extremely motivating.
2. There is power in prayer.
3. Faith renders cancer a win-win.
4. You can learn to manage stress.

ACTIONABLE HOPE

It's time to get real about your habits. What lifestyle changes would help you in your wellness plan?

What affirmations would strengthen the beliefs you need for your recovery? You can do a search on the internet for lots of affirmations revolving around health and wellness. You can write your own, too.

Focus on this thought: I have today, and today I am a survivor. (Repeat it over and over in your mind.)

What other beliefs should you affirm to prepare you for this battle?

Do you believe in the power of prayer? If so, how consistent are you with your prayer time?

When can you protect some time in your day for prayer?

Download an app or listen to a video of guided meditation.

Practice for fifteen minutes every day.

CHAPTER 8

BELIEVE IT OR NOT

Where there is great love, there are always miracles.

—WILLA CATHER

When I was growing up, holidays were magical. No school and gifts! What a combination. As a new parent, the joy of the holidays multiplied tenfold! My son had his first birthday party, and I was excited to enjoy Christmas with him. The shopping and decorating were in full swing. Meeting deadlines at work was a struggle because my to-do list was a mile long and my brain was at the North Pole. Then the phone rang.

"Do you have a son named Nicholas?" I didn't recognize the voice and I wondered who this was that knew my baby's name. I must have told her I did because she continued, "You need to come to the hospital as quickly as possible. Your baby is here but it's not good. He doesn't have much time. Hurry!"

The days before cell phones were different. Now we have constant contact. That drive to the hospital was silent. I had no idea what happened. I had dropped him off at the little farm daycare that morning. He was perfectly healthy. I did not care one bit about speed limits or police. I drove faster than I had ever driven before. My mind was full of questions. What in the world was going on?

As I ran through the doors into the hospital, I saw Julia, the daycare provider. She tried to hug me and say she was sorry, but a nurse ran over, confirmed my identity, and then led me to a gurney in triage. There was my pale little baby not moving at all swarmed by scurrying scrubs. "What happened?" My words were hardly audible as I could barely push breath through my vocal cords.

A doctor introduced himself and then started to explain. "He ingested kerosene." I was confused. How does a baby ingest kerosene? He started drawing me a diagram of his heart and his lungs, and my head was just swimming. I put my hand over his pen, and he finally looked in my eyes and realized I was overwhelmed. "Is he going to make it?" That's all I wanted to know.

"I don't know," he sighed. The moment was interrupted by somebody telling him the helicopter was ready. He told me that parents aren't allowed to fly but that he was personally flying to Johns Hopkins with my baby. By this time my husband arrived, and we were allowed to kiss baby Nicholas on the cheek before they rushed him away. As we hurried to the car, the helicopter lifted into the air, taking my breath away.

Ninety minutes. No cell phones. Will our son still be alive when we get there? Silence. Waves of various emotions flooded my mind. When fear retreated, anger crashed in. The miles seemed endless.

The daycare decision was difficult. I interviewed several and had him in the care of another place for a couple of weeks, but I wasn't satisfied because I didn't feel Nick was getting enough attention. Julia was referred to me, and I loved the fact that she lived on a little farm. It was a licensed daycare, and she didn't have any other children she was caring for at that time. Nicholas would have all of her attention. I envisioned them going out in the mornings and singing "Old MacDonald" as they looked at the chickens and goats. I never imagined she would have him shut in her bedroom while she was vacuuming in the hall. I certainly never dreamed she would have a decorative kerosene candle on the bottom shelf of a bookshelf. Not even in my worst nightmare could I see him drinking it like a bottle. That's what happened, though.

Nick survived the flight, and I took up residence in his room in the pediatric intensive care unit. Time just seemed to freeze for days. It's amazing how it flies by so quickly that your head spins, but when it comes to a screeching grind, it's just torture. A ventilator was breathing for him. Julia had enough foresight to bring the bottle of kerosene to the hospital, so it sat by the door staring at me. I tried to ignore it, but it taunted me until I asked for it to be taken away. It angered me. The scent of the gas seeping out of his pores hovered like vultures flying around him. It gagged me.

The Ronald McDonald House gave us a place where we could sleep and shower along with a stocked kitchen. There sure wasn't much sleeping or eating for me, but I am forever grateful for such an amazing charity. Days and nights just blended together, each an extension of time that didn't seem to have a point.

Eventually one of the doctors interrupted my endless thoughts and prayers to inform me, "It's time." They had told me they couldn't induce vomiting because Nick's lungs would not survive and he would die, so the only thing they could do was wait until the gas escaped his body on its own. The doctor said it was time to shut down the ventilator.

"Is he going to breathe on his own?" I demanded to know. The look on the doctor's face wasn't reassuring at all. In fact, it was quite blank. "Well, is he?" There was no way to know for sure what would happen. Best-case scenario, he would breathe and then we'd figure out further complications from there. The worst-case scenario was written all over the doctor's face. I shuttered.

Tears streamed down my face as I held his little hand. The room went quiet. I hadn't even noticed the sound the machine was making until it ceased. Time stopped. I didn't breathe. Nobody in the room breathed. Nobody moved. Everything was just frozen, until it happened. His little chest expanded. We all saw it. We all heard it. I collapsed.

The days that followed were full of tests, and my active little baby started coming back to life. Before I knew it, we were being discharged. I tracked down the doctor in the halls of the hospital to tell him thank you before we left. I will never forget his response. He humbly said, "Don't thank me. I didn't do anything. There wasn't anything I *could* do. There is no medical reason for Nicholas to be alive. He is an anomaly. Don't thank me. Thank God."

Those words lingered in my head on the long drive home. The sun was going down and all the pretty lights outlined houses and trees. Everything looked so festive. I forgot it was December. As we pulled onto our street, I was relieved to see our home, and I hadn't even noticed how strangely dark the houses were on our street in contrast to all of the other bright houses I saw along the way. As I was getting the baby out of the car, I saw a neighbor open her door, and immediately she flipped her Christmas lights on. I smiled and then noticed another neighbor who did the same thing. One by one, the houses lit up, and the neighborhood twinkled happily. The first neighbor came out onto the sidewalk to tell me they had all been waiting to turn their lights on that season until little St. Nicholas came home. It was a miracle, plain and simple.

Do you believe in miracles? I don't know how I would have answered that question prior to that Christmas. As I moved through the process of cancer, I started watching videos about miracles. I didn't care if they were cancer-related or not—it didn't matter. I just wanted to surround myself with miraculous stories. Later I learned the term "spontaneous remission" and discovered a whole book about all these cancer patients and their documented recoveries. It's called *Radical Remission* by Kelly Turner.[2]

There's another book that challenges the notion that spontaneous remission is rare. Perhaps it is more prevalent than we realize, suggests Jeffrey Rediger, MD, in *Cured: The Life-Changing Science of Spontaneous Healing*.

EXPECT A MIRACLE

When we think of miracles, we naturally think big. My little baby Nicholas was a huge miracle. Every spontaneous remission is an incredible miracle. I'm sure you and all of the rest of us in the Ovary Jones club would love a spontaneous remission miracle. Should we hope for a miracle? Dare we expect a miracle?

---

2   Kelly A. Turner, *Radical Remission: Surviving Cancer against All Odds* (New York: HarperOne, 2014).

A friend called telling me about Patrick, our mutual friend, who was racing around the Autobahn in a Lamborghini four months after he was told he had two months to live. My heart melted with joy as I imagined the smile plastered on Patrick's face and the exhilaration he was feeling. Patrick had always dreamed of experiencing the speed of such an impressive masterpiece. Is Patrick the living proof of a miracle? What if Patrick becomes a winged warrior tomorrow? Is his miracle nullified? A lot of people would have gone home to wait for their pending expiration date upon hearing such a grim diagnosis. Not Patrick. Ever since his diagnosis, he has been checking things off of his bucket list like it's his job.

Truth be told, every day is a miracle. When we get in the habit of expecting and looking for miracles, we start noticing them. If ever I start to doubt, I just place my hand on my port just below my right collar bone. Modern medicine might not have every cure, but it sure is full of miracles. The human body is a miracle. I thank God every morning for the gift of a new day, fully understanding I am not entitled to another minute. I didn't *earn* it. I expect a new day. I plan for a future. I'm also pleasantly surprised every time the morning sun creeps in and kisses my cheeks.

You've been given the gift of today. Sure, it comes with challenges. It's not perfect. Maybe it's even raining. It's yours, though. Yours to curse or yours to appreciate. The gift is yours, but it comes with a choice.

Search for the hidden miracles that are more subtle. I believe we overlook these gems every day. We get so fixated looking for the big miracles that we miss the opportunity to celebrate the frequency of the daily miracles. Is life a coincidence or a miracle?

Have we grown weary of these miracles, or does our life have to be *perfect* to appreciate them? When did the amazement of the world around us wear off? Perhaps it's time to fall back in love with being alive. Maybe cancer makes us simpleminded, but I'm more blown away now than ever before by more than just the seven natural wonders of the world, including:

- Cherry blossoms every spring
- The beauty of the setting sun
- The birth of every baby
- The change of every season
- Love
- The fact that you have been breathing since you were born
- The healing of our skin after an incision
- The growth of infants to toddlers to teens to adults
- How your heart has been beating around the clock since you were born

- The fact that cells that make up the largest organ of your body, your skin, are replaced every two to three weeks
- The fact that dogs are miracles with paws, providing unconditional love without holding grudges
- Hair that grows back
- The kiss of sunlight on my face every single morning that I get to be alive

This list could continue endlessly, but you get the point. Rejoice and appreciate all of the things that perhaps you once took for granted. I know I did.

Remember what it was like to discover something for the first time? Maybe you were awestruck. There are amazing things in the world around us. Surely, we haven't discovered them all. Perhaps it's time to be on the lookout for things that marvel us. There are miracles all around us. Let's find them!

LIFE-PROLONGING TAKEAWAYS

1. Expect a miracle.
2. Greet each day as a pleasant surprise.
3. We can still be awestruck every day.

ACTIONABLE HOPE

Watch videos on miracles.

Fill your mind up with positive inspiration every day.

Keep identifying things you are grateful for every day.

Find a miracle to marvel every day.

CHAPTER 9

SCANXIETY

Extreme fear can neither fight nor fly.

—WILLIAM SHAKESPEARE

Fear is not a way of life. We can't live waiting for the next shoe to drop. Nonetheless, waiting for test results every week, or every six months, or every year can be heart-wrenching. Often cancer requires multiple battles.

As members of the Ovary Jones society, we have to discover coping mechanisms to deal with worry, fear, hopelessness, feelings of overwhelm, and the fact that we are not always in control of cancer. All of what we thought we knew is now vastly different. Our perspective has forever shifted.

One of the best things we can do comes from Socrates: "Know thyself." Everybody is different. One of the questions you will likely be asked at every visit is about your mental health. Depression can show up with different signs and symptoms. Talk to your doctors. They are on your team.

PUCKER FACTOR

One of my friends served in Iraq. He talked about traveling on the Baghdad Airport Road, also known as Route Irish and the most dangerous road in the world. The stretch of highway seven-and-a-half miles long connects the Green Zone (the international zone of Baghdad) and the airport. He and his soldiers were well aware of the grave danger from either side of the road along the way. I can only imagine what those men and women thought about for almost ten minutes as they traveled down a highway notorious for random shootings, suicide bombers, and roadside bombs. As my friend so adequately summed it up, the pucker factor is high when you go outside the wire. (If you are unfamiliar with military jargon, *pucker factor* is the adrenaline response to a crisis, and it literally refers to tightening the buttocks due to extreme fear.) For them, it's the mission that gets them through. That is what they focus on. He said you override the anxiety because you're on a mission, which is more important than any individual. He said, "We were willing to lay our lives down for the bigger picture. We're going home one way or another." As he remembered those treks, he seemed to relive the emotions and even sighed as he recounted seeing Baghdad International Airport. He said it was always a relief because you knew you were safe.

Maybe we can't completely take away the pucker factor of scanxiety just like those soldiers couldn't erase the pucker factor as they drove along that dangerous stretch. I don't know of anybody who would describe those marines as weak, so we have to remember that being afraid is not being weak. Perhaps the best we can do is focus on the mission, which is to discover what is happening in our bodies so we can take action. Courage isn't the absence or removal of fear; it is instead the choice to act in spite of fear.

Loretta LaRoche is an internationally renowned author and stress-management consultant who advocates humor, optimism, and resiliency as coping mechanisms for stress. She said something that I've never forgotten and I think of every single time I go for a scan. I hope it helps you as much as it helps me. She said, "If you think the worst and get the worst, you suffer twice. If you think the best and get the worst, you only suffer once." Let's not suffer more than we have to.

THE POWER OF VAN

Some words have many meanings and some things are hard to put into words. One thing cancer patients get used to is blood draws. My team kept close tabs on my platelets. They always asked me to rate my fatigue on a scale of 1 to 10. Then they would ask me about shortness of breath. Fatigue and shortness of breath were new to me. I didn't know what they felt like and I didn't know how to describe how I felt. They were looking at my numbers, which didn't mean anything to me, and asking me to describe how I felt because according to my numbers, I must have been pretty wiped out. I remember one nurse asking if I wanted her to ask about getting a blood transfusion.

Blood transfusion? That sounded scary. Even before the COVID-19 pandemic, I preferred to keep to myself. I cringed anytime I saw anybody drink out of the same straw as somebody else. Social distancing was not a big challenge for me. I didn't really understand what all was involved in a blood transfusion. Do they take all of your blood out of one side of your body while pumping somebody else's blood into you on the other side? I imagined some sort of 1950s low-budget sci-fi movie. The thought of somebody else's blood in my body creeped me out. I rejected the idea without asking a single question.

A few more weeks dragged by. I could barely take the dog out. Moving was cumbersome. I needed multiple naps throughout the day. My quality of life was dismal, and I wondered if this was how it was going to be from now on. The nurse approached me again about a transfusion. She said my numbers were critically low. I still cringed, but I asked her about the safety of it and what it entailed. She explained there are risks with everything, but she said my numbers were so low that she was confident the benefits would be substantial. Reluctantly, I agreed.

On the morning of my transfusion, I practically crawled into the hospital. The West Penn Hospital in Pittsburgh is a large academic medical center that has been around since the mid-1800s. Because I spent so much time there walking the halls for weeks when I was first diagnosed, I know the facility well. It is not a short walk from the parking garage to the elevators. Even though I was more familiar with the procedure, it was still foreign to me and the pucker factor was high. I was nervous.

One of the things that always comforted me was thinking about my grandmother, all of the other Ovary Jones mavericks, and one little boy in particular. His name is Van and he is the son of Ron Alford, who is pretty much a rock star at Southwestern Consulting. Everybody has great respect for Ron because he is a rare, can-do visionary with an unbreakable spirit. He's an achiever who leads with conviction because he strongly believes success and enduring joy comes from principle-centered living. Then Van was diagnosed with leukemia. Cancer always sucks, but when it messes with children it takes cruelty to the next level.

A cancer diagnosis will test anybody's foundation. Watching this family pull together to rise above was inspiring. Ron and his wife, Desiree, Van and his twin brother, PK, and their little sister, Hartley, demonstrated how to get stronger through fire. Instead of allowing cancer the ability to introduce discord in the family, their bond was strengthened through Van and multiplied by the power of God.

When I prepared for tests that made me uneasy, and this transfusion in particular, I prayed to be brave like Van. During every test, I would think if a child can be brave, surely I could too. Van became my hero. That's what it means to tap into the spirit of Ovary Jones. I've never met Van. He lives on the other side of the country. Cancer has brought all of us together on the same battlefield. It unifies us even if it is the only common denominator we share. You are not alone. By the way, when I heard after three years Van was in remission, I cried like a baby. Happy tears for a hero I've never met.

It turns out, blood transfusions are miracles! Instantly I had more energy. I struggled into the hospital, and I practically skipped like a schoolgirl all the way out. It was the most amazing phenomenon, and had I not experienced it myself, I'm not sure I could believe it. Other women can go spend the day at a spa, but send me to the blood bank! I had a new lease on life and more energy than I had in a year. It turns out, sometimes what we fear never actually happens. We worry for nothing! If I wouldn't have taken action, I would not have been blessed with that incredible reward. Don't let fear stop you!

STRESS-ERCISE

You know there are going to be more tests and stressful days ahead, so it's smart to plan ahead. Develop techniques today for the stressful tomorrows that will come our way. While your stress is not acute, practice techniques that will help on *those* days—when the pucker factor is high. The more I read, the more I'm convinced of the negative effects of too much stress in our lives. Being busy is highly regaled like a badge of honor in society, perhaps to our detriment. Few people make time to relax every day, but even short periods of downtime free from electronics and the hustle and bustle of the day can be helpful. When we want to improve our physical resilience, we exercise every day. We start with a few pushups, and gradually we work to be able to do more. When it comes to improving our mental resilience, we have to work at it every day too. We practice the big three every day like we practice pushups (affirmations, prayer, and meditation discussed in the previous chapter). There are other things we can add to our daily routine to reduce stress and improve our grit.

What do you enjoy doing that is solely for you? I'm going to guess that was a challenging question to answer. There are so many wonderful ways we can reduce stress, but too often we forget because we get so caught up providing for other people. I remember when the diagnosis was fresh how frustrated I was because I didn't have time for cancer. I was too busy, and I'm sure that wasn't serving me well at all. Perhaps your body was trying to get your attention.

Carve out time for you every day. Find something you enjoy doing. Even if you can only find thirty minutes, there's so much you could do. Take a walk. Close your eyes and just relax. Listen to your favorite song. Write in a journal or jot down a few things you're grateful for. Turn some music on and bust a move. Listen to a comedian or a motivational speaker on a podcast or YouTube. If at all possible, find ways to move your body.

Try to find a little longer period of time for things you enjoy once or twice a week. Perhaps then you can take a painting class or do something artistic. Maybe you play an instrument or sing. Go to a yoga class. Take a bubble bath. Did you know they make coloring books for grown-ups? Perhaps you could make thank-you cards, which will help you tap into your creative side and focus on gratitude at the same time.

When I was freshly diagnosed, I remember thinking, "This is it? You've got to be kidding me?! I worked my tail off my whole life, and this is it?" I don't want to have those thoughts again. You might feel a little guilty shutting the world out and taking time for you. You are not being selfish, and there's no reason to feel guilty. You've probably been giving your whole life, so think of it as giving yourself the gift of healing.

The idea that we have to learn how to relax sounds strange. Many of us do, however, need to learn the art of relaxation. Our body isn't built for chronic stress. Relax every day, get plenty of sleep, enjoy fruits and vegetables, drink water, laugh, exercise, and socialize. That sounds like a pretty sweet life! It just takes a little planning, which I'm sure you're up for.

When it is time for another scan, just go. We all know early detection is key, so we don't want to procrastinate. While you're waiting for the results, choose any of the aforementioned activities that you've been practicing every day in between your scans.

Many people have pondered our response to the things that scare us. C. S. Lewis wrote the following way back in 1948 in his essay "On Living in an Atomic Age." We could easily replace the word *bomb* with COVID-19, cancer, and many other things we fear.

> This is the first point to be made: and the first action to be taken is to pull ourselves together. If we are all going to be destroyed by an atomic bomb, let that bomb when it comes find us doing sensible and human things—praying, working, teaching, reading, listening to music, bathing the children, playing tennis, chatting to our friends over a pint and a game of darts—not huddled together like frightened sheep and thinking about bombs. They may break our bodies (a microbe can do that) but they need not dominate our minds.[3]

---

3 C. S. Lewis and Walter Hooper, *Present Concerns* (London: Fount Paperbacks, 1987).

LIFE-PROLONGING TAKEAWAYS

1. Fear is not a way of life.
2. If you think the worst and get the worst, you suffer twice. If you think the best and get the worst, you only suffer once.
3. Other women can go to the spa, but send me to the blood bank!

ACTIONABLE HOPE

What *can* you do?

Build a puzzle, make handmade cards, write a poem, take a walk, sing, dance, read.

Learn something new. Most of us have access to the internet or books. What is something new you would like to learn? (Instead of focusing on the things you can't do right now, think of things you *can* do.)

CHAPTER 10

WHAT'S WEIGHING YOU DOWN?

Anger is an acid that can do more harm to the vessel in which it is stored than to anything on which it is poured.

—MARK TWAIN

We're supposed to do this together. Research actually proves solitude is deadly. I mentioned earlier that conflicting emotions can't reside in one heart. Your heart cannot be full of happiness and anger at the same time. It is binary. Either/or. In other words, you choose. What are you focusing on? I beg you to zoom in on all the little things you have to be grateful for.

Let go of the rest. Release any negative feelings you are clenching like a security blanket simply because they are so familiar to you. You'll notice that it feels like releasing the shackles of an anchor wrapped around your feet and swimming to the surface for fresh air. I only know because I did it. I had to for my own sanity. Let the negativity drop with a thud. You don't need it. You will feel lighter. You can't solve all of the injustices of the world. You can only work on the reflection in your mirror. Holding onto negative emotions for an extended period of time is not serving you. It certainly isn't hurting cancer. It isn't hurting anybody else whom you might be resenting. It's hurting you! Let go. You can do it.

Sometimes it is a challenge. I didn't say it's easy. I'm not even suggesting you somehow stop all negative thoughts and feelings. That's impossible. Let them come in like a wave. Recognize them, experience them, face them. Stare them down if you have to. When you are ready, exhale them. It is a process, and like any process, it takes time. We can't just ignore our feelings and hope they go away. We have to deal with them. Then the healing process can begin. We can start to replace them with gratitude or something positive. As you practice, you'll get better and the waves won't come as often.

You have to make a conscious effort. Effort means work. Work is not easy by definition, but you can do it. The goal is to release any grudges or resentments you might have toward anybody or anything. Again, not easy. Trust me, I know! I think of it like losing weight. Usually we gain weight slowly. (Unless you gain it like I did on the steroids, which was ridiculously fast.) It usually creeps up on us. Maybe you've done what I've done in the past and made a New Year's resolution to lose ten pounds. If you're anything like me, by June you have fifteen pounds to go. Resolving our resentments is similar. Too often, we've been carrying grudges and resentments with us for many years. We can't expect they're just going to go away because we decide we want them to. Like losing weight, it takes time. We have to break the habit of holding on to resentments and replace it with something that will serve us better.

Maybe you have held onto a grudge so long that you forget exactly why it started in the first place. Maybe that story has taken on a life of its own over the years. One of my friends was struggling with this, so we spent some time writing down exactly what each grievance was, whom she was holding the grudge over, why she was hurt by it and the feelings she experienced because of each incidence, and what role she might have had in the situations. She was able to get all of the negative emotions off of her chest and onto a piece of paper where she could see them much more logically. When she was ready, we had a fire and we watched that paper and those negative emotions burn. She decided if any of those people popped into her mind again, she would remind herself how much stronger she is because of them.

KINDRED SPIRITS

Five years ago, my best friend in the world was ripped away from me by an evil, maniacal creature who happened to be her husband of twenty years and the father of her three children. Dana Wilson Miller was the Thelma to my Louise. (I actually called her "T" and she called me "L," but of course we weren't planning to drive off a cliff or anything.) Dana could make me laugh like nobody else on the planet.

We were in constant communication, texting from sunup to sundown eight days a week. We wrapped Christmas presents "together" every Christmas Eve till wee hours in the morning via texting or talking on the phone. Birthdays, holidays, and all the ordinary days in between were shared experiences.

I was always a bit of a guarded person, much more apt to listen than talk, especially about myself. There was no hiding with Dana though. She wasn't shy or reserved at all, and just about every thought that popped into her head escaped from her mouth. Anything she ever wanted to know, she asked. At first, I didn't like her nosey nature, but that didn't stop her from asking anyway. Eventually I learned to trust her, and we had the most authentic and transparent friendship I've ever had with anybody.

Dana loved to cook, shop, decorate, and drink wine. I let her excel in all of those things because she was more competitive than me and I benefited from all her talents anyway. What we had in common was a sharp and quick-witted sarcasm that bonded us together like superglue. Together we laughed—at each other, at ourselves, and at life in general—which is rich with humor for anyone paying attention.

When you are born in the suburbs of Pittsburgh, you're wrapped in a Myron Cope Terrible Towel in the delivery room. Parents from Pittsburgh hold their babies like footballs, and the lullaby they sing at night as they rock their future fans to sleep is "Renegade," the anthem played at every Steelers home game. The story they repeat to their toddler on their knee is "The Immaculate Reception," which never gets old. Dana and I were Pittsburgh born and raised, which means we grew up with champions.

She usually invited us to watch the games at her house, and since the kids were all friends, they loved to go. My oldest son, Nick, loved her cooking more than mine, and she thought that was the greatest. He kept complimenting her and she kept serving him. They both loved it. He truly thought of her like his second mother. One particular Sunday I asked the usual obligatory question, "What can I bring?" I expected her to say, "Nothing," because that was her usual response, perhaps because she knew my culinary skills, or lack thereof. This time she told me to bring buffalo chicken dip. Like all talented tailgaters, that was a dish I could make in my sleep, which I wish I would have done.

Instead time got the best of me and we got home from church late, and before I knew it, the time was 12:55. Five minutes before game time and the choice was either miss the kickoff or skip the dip. I was born red, white, blue, black, and gold. Of course, I threw everything into a bag and got the kids in the car because the game was about to start! I will never forget the confused look on her face when she opened the door. The very first thing she asked was, "Where's the dip?" All I could do was grin and hold up the bag.

"WHO DOES THAT?" I could tell she was a little angry, but fortunately she was also humored. We made it together. (Okay, she mostly made it.) She never let me live that down. She also never asked me to bring the dip again. That was a bonus.

It wasn't fair that she was taken away. I was angry. I wanted her to make fun of me for taking a sack of ingredients to her house instead of the prepared dish she was expecting. I wanted her to ask me all her endless detail questions about all the tests the coats were running, how much it was costing me, and how everything felt. I especially wanted her to try to tell me how I looked just as beautiful with a shiny bald head as I did with my long locks while keeping a straight face.

I needed her but she wasn't there. I wasn't the only one who needed her these past few years. Her kids needed her as they graduated high school and went off to college. Her parents needed her. Her brothers and her many, many friends needed her. Honestly, I was spitting angry at her husband, not only for robbing Dana of her life and all of us from her love, but also for cowardly taking his own life. I didn't have anybody to yell at and there wasn't anybody I could hate. I wanted justice for Dana. I dreamed about his day in court. My testimony. Looking at him in the eye and pointing to him, the guilty one. I longed to watch him try to shuffle to his forever cinder-home as he tripped over his shackles.

Instead I got to discover what the world was like without laughter, love, and a friendship that comes around once in a lifetime, if we're lucky. My phone died with her. It didn't wake me up in the morning. It didn't keep me up at night. It punished me with silence because she no longer sent me a never-ending string of texts. Time moved on only because it doesn't stand still. I didn't want it to.

This was the pent-up bitterness and resentment I needed to release. My best friend was murdered in cold blood by her husband. She was shot three times in the back in their gorgeous home where they were raising their children. Forgiving the unforgivable and accepting an unspoken apology are challenging but healthy endeavors.

What resides in your heart? Conflicting emotions don't mix; it's one or the other. Love or hate. Joy or sadness. Happiness or anger. Resentment or forgiveness. As I practiced gratitude for experiencing a rare friendship rich with trust and vulnerability, I let go of the hatred I was clinging to toward an evil ghost, the memory of a cowardly man.

As always, I cherish Dana's memories and I long to make it to London so I can visit our dear mutual friend. I look forward to talking about Dana and exchanging memories with somebody who knew and loved her too.

COMMUNITY IS CRITICAL

Amazingly, as I exhaled my resentment, I found room in my heart for new friends and, to my astonishment, I suddenly had a whole club of people to talk to, and we have a lot in common.

Don't be afraid to talk to people when you are getting treatments. That's how I met Beth. We happened to be infusion chair neighbors during one of our treatments. I couldn't see her because of a half-drawn curtain between the chairs, but I heard her ring a little bell. Within seconds every chemo-hanging angel on the unit was by her side. I was worried for my neighbor and said a little prayer. Her rescue party disbanded, and I could hear her talking to her husband.

I stood up and dragged my pole over so I could see her. "How did you make all those people move so quickly? I don't have a bell. Why don't I have a bell?" We both laughed. I am so blessed to have my chemo buddy Beth and her husband, Cecil, in my life now. We would touch base after our treatments to check in on each other. We compared notes and side effects on the drugs we were both on. Everybody needs a Beth! I'm so glad she rang that bell!

If you can, go to support groups, but not all groups are created equal. Beth had some experiences that left her more depressed than encouraged. There's a big difference between lifting each other up and having a pity party. Find the groups that empower you.

Allow your friends and family in on this journey (as long as they are positive people) for your benefit but for theirs as well. This is not a time to be aloof, stoic, or prideful. You've been giving and giving your whole life. It's time to receive. Allow others the opportunity of sharing this challenge with you.

LIFE-PROLONGING TAKEAWAYS

1. Happiness and anger cannot reside in the same space.
2. Grudges are unnecessary self-inflicting pain.
3. We are stronger together.
4. Find the groups that lift you up.

ACTIONABLE HOPE

Dump resentment, bitterness, and any grudges you might be carrying.

Make friends. Talk to people in treatment with you or at support groups.

Write out grievances you might have toward anyone. What exactly did each person do? How did you feel about it? What role did you have in each situation? Are there any notable patterns? What lessons did these situations teach you that you can be thankful for? Destroy the paper when you are ready to.

CHAPTER 11

TOGETHER WE BOX

Alone we can do so little; together we can do so much.

—HELEN KELLER

When you can, get back to giving back. There's nothing like volunteering or engaging in an altruistic endeavor to express compassion and gratitude for our extended play. There certainly isn't any shortage of people who need our help or our time. It always feels good to plug into something bigger than any individual. You will learn a lot from your journey that can help newly diagnosed members of our society.

This is truly why my daughter and I started *Together We Box*, a monthly subscription care package full of actionable hope. There were so many people who wanted to help me in the beginning of my journey, but they didn't know how. Dr. Sarah Miller told me one day she gets asked all the time from friends and family, "What can I do?" We wanted to help those on the sidelines by giving them something they can do. The monthly boxes are full of encouragement and ideas that my fellow Ovary Jones sisters can do every day to develop mental toughness for this fight. Of course, there are also things that are fun and some of the new "friendlier" products I've been discovering packed in every box.

It was hard getting out, and for once in my life I didn't want to go shopping. It went from my favorite pastime to a chore in a hurry. So now we get to do a little shopping for our Ovary Jones sorority sisters because we believe warriors appreciate luxury too.

Kenzie and I literally set out to change the way the cancer battle is fought by strengthening the mental game with monthly care packages and online resources full of encouragement, empowerment, and actionable hope. We pack every box with grit and grace, and love and laughter.

It's not that I have a new lease on life, because honestly my life doesn't resemble my B.C. (before cancer) life very much at all. It's a new life. Sure, I fortunately have the same cast of core characters, but now I have a lot of new friends and the Ovary Jones club whom I care so much about. I'm blessed with a new sense of belonging in a community I might not have chosen, but still I'm grateful for. While I'm still not able to convincingly shout out, "I'm thankful for my cancer,"

I will confess I'm progressing toward that end. I've come a long way, and so will you. So, let me repeat what I said in the very beginning: Welcome to the club! You can do it!

LIFE-PROLONGING TAKEAWAYS

1. We feel alive when we give back.
2. Your life will likely change through this.
3. You can do this.

ACTIONABLE HOPE

Write a note of encouragement to somebody today.

Find a way to pay it forward.

CONCLUSION

To me, every hour of the day and night is an unspeakably perfect miracle.

—WALT WHITMAN

Take a deep breath, sunshine. You can do this! I'm thrilled to share that my dad is still walking with N.E.D (No Evidence of Disease) and doing well, as am I. Beth is too. In fact, so is the neighbor, Paul. This can change at any moment for any of us, but that is okay. You are going to learn so much about yourself, about others, and about life.

BEAUTY IN CANCER

I'm an optimist to an admitted fault. Sometimes my head is so far in the clouds, my feet aren't touching the ground. Added with a seemingly never-ending supply of naivety, it can be a problem or a source of humor. If you ever had a baby, you probably remember all of the anticipation and excitement leading up to the big day. I remember packing my hospital bag. I had such a cute coming-home outfit for our new addition. I also had my favorite jeans and a cute top for me. Mind you, they were not maternity jeans at all. I don't know why I just expected that after I had the baby, my body would just magically return to normal. While I laugh about that now, the same thing happened with my cancer treatments.

Perhaps you're like me and you think everything will go back to the way it was before you had cancer. Truth is, there will be things that are different. I thought when I finished chemotherapy, I wouldn't be as fatigued. I thought I would have all of the energy I used to have. I thought the weight would just fall off just like it didn't do when I had my babies. I thought my hair would grow back much faster.

Reality is different. Getting back to the way you were before cancer takes work, and even then, it will likely be different. I used to have a normal-looking stomach—not six-pack abs—but I was relatively fit. When the dust settled from all my body went through, my stomach was oddly shaped. It always looked like I had shoplifted something that I was hiding in my shirt. My clothes didn't fit the same. I couldn't do all of the things I used to easily do.

It was a tradeoff. My body was weaker, but my mind was

much stronger. Yoga has helped tremendously, and I've been gritting through more exercise. The weight might all come off eventually. I did discover the miracle of Spanx. The scars will always be there. The radiation tattoos will never go away. Things are different.

This experience is going to change you. You are not going to come out of it quite the same. Lean into it. Resolve to come through this mentally stronger. Understand that the lessons you will learn come at a price. Decide that the education is worth it. This is an opportunity if you choose to see it as such. Hit the reset button and create a new future—a new you. Only then will the new and improved version of you be able to see… there is beauty in cancer. Perhaps this was my most surprising revelation of all. The late, great motivational speaker, Zig Ziglar, figured this out way before me when he said, "Difficult roads often lead to beautiful destinations." Finally, I agree.

Beth believes she's a better person because of her journey. She said she wasn't where she wanted to be spiritually. In her words, she said, "I'm glad God picked me to go through this because it has made me a stronger Christian and it has made me a better person. I'm more compassionate now. It made me grow in a good way and I am better because of it." (You might have to trust me on this, but good really can come from this!)

We are all thankful for the miracles we see in every day.

Like everybody in the Ovary Jones club, we know tomorrow isn't promised, so we appreciate each day as the gift that it is. Being present and in the moment comes naturally now. In fact, things that used to be stressful don't cause nearly as much panic as they did in the dark age before cancer. We all feel a bit enlightened.

P.S. I LOVE YOU

Ready for the best part? We have a *Together We Box* line of natural, luxury soaps and lotions for the subscription boxes. The line came about because I was determined to find bubble baths, lotions, and all the fun stuff that are not laced with harmful toxins. Surely, I could find products that work, are safer, and feel fantastic too! One of our fan favorites is our P.S. I Love You. The scent is amazing. It makes me so happy that women love the soaps, lotions, and scrubs in this particular scent because this one happens to be very near and dear to my heart.

Early on, I asked my doctors if I would live long enough to meet my grandchildren. "Probably not," was the answer. My stubborn daughter taught me when she was a toddler that *probably not* means *maybe* and *maybe* could mean *yes*. That's all I needed to hear. Turns out my daughter got her determination honestly.

What I'm over the moon to announce is the birth of my

granddaughter, Paisley Sage. She is the P.S. in P.S. I Love You. She has me wrapped around her tiny little pinky. Of course, P.S. I Love You is our number-one fan favorite. I guess I shouldn't be surprised at all. MiMi loves her little miracle…she is breathtaking!

ALL OF THE LIFE-PROLONGING TAKEAWAYS

1. Mindset impacts outcomes.
2. You are part of the Ovary Jones club of brave mavericks who came before us.
3. There's no better time than now to be diagnosed with cancer.
4. You can still be happy.
5. Good can come from bad.
6. The healthcare professionals are on *your* team…you're the captain, and you pick the team.
7. Take an active role in your recovery.
8. Love is powerfully motivating.
9. Cancer happens to the whole family.
10. If one survived, so can you…if none have survived, be the first.
11. Nobody has a crystal ball.
12. Take this journey one step at a time.
13. Assume victory. Hope is everything.
14. Mental toughness is learned and requires practice.
15. Gratitude must be our daily focus.
16. Some weirdos are thankful for cancer; I'm determined to be one of them.

17. Feelings follow action.
18. Courage resides on the other side of fear.
19. Your mind is essential to your recovery.
20. Disappointment comes when expectations don't match reality.
21. You have been given the gift of perspective.
22. Your mind is powerful.
23. Words matter.
24. Don't believe everything you think.
25. What you look for, you will find. Seek out happiness.
26. Lunch with friends is healing.
27. The mental game has to be fought first before healing can take place.
28. Protect yourself from the ignorance of well-meaning people.
29. Beliefs are powerful.
30. Programming is your responsibility.
31. Change is a decision.
32. We live in a toxic world.
33. Exercise reduces fatigue.
34. A cancer diagnosis can be extremely motivating.
35. There is power in prayer.
36. Faith renders cancer a win-win.
37. You can learn to manage stress.
38. Expect a miracle.
39. Greet each day as a pleasant surprise.
40. We can still be awestruck every day.
41. Fear is not a way of life.

42. If you think the worst and get the worst, you suffer twice. If you think the best and get the worst, you only suffer once.

43. Other women can go to the spa, but send me to the blood bank!

44. Happiness and anger cannot reside in the same space.

45. Grudges are unnecessary self-inflicting pain.

46. We are stronger together.

47. Find the groups that lift you up.

48. We feel alive when we give back.

49. Your life will likely change through this.

50. You can do this.

ACTIONABLE HOPE

Join our Facebook online fight club!

Share your journal of the lessons you learn in your journey. Adversity is a humbling teacher, but the lessons she teaches are beautiful, nonetheless.

APPENDIX A

Keep reading!

Radical Remission by Kelly Turner

Do you believe in miracles? I don't know how I would have answered that question prior to the Christmas when my son defied all odds and lived, shocking the local medical community where we lived. As I moved through the process of cancer, I started watching videos about miracles. I didn't care if they were cancer-related or not—it didn't matter. I just wanted to surround myself with miraculous stories. Later I learned the term "spontaneous remission" and discovered a whole book about all these cancer patients and their documented recoveries. I highly recommend it.

Cured: The Life-Changing Science of Spontaneous Healing by Jeffrey Rediger, MD

Another book that challenges the notion that spontaneous remission is rare. Perhaps it is more prevalent than we realize?

The Silver Lining: A Supportive and Insightful Guide to Breast Cancer by Hollye Jacobs, RN, MS, MSW

While I didn't have breast cancer, I did stumble upon this book, and it has a lot of practical suggestions on everything from how to tell people about your diagnosis (especially children) to what to pack when you go in for surgery. The author talked about 'roid rage (the intense feelings of anger brought on by pre-chemotherapy steroids) and chemo sobby (tears at the drop of a hat brought on by the chemo drugs). I didn't really have the first but I certainly got emotional way more than I ever had before. I remember being in a work meeting just after my last chemo treatment, and every little thing brought tears to my eyes. I'm better now, but I did learn to just go with the flow and embrace it. The guide would be helpful as you learn all the new terminology and you figure out all the tests and the ins and outs of the cancer patient's world. It really is like learning a new language, but soon you'll be talking the talk and discovering it's a process—long and grueling, yes—but a process nonetheless.

How to Make Disease Disappear by Dr. Rangan Chatterjee

There are so many different diets out there, and it seems like every year there's a new exercise fad. This is the book that made sense to me and shaped my thinking when it comes to a sustainable lifestyle. It is easy to follow and has practical, encompassing ideas about nutrition, stress, and exercise that have made a huge difference in the lives of his patients.

What to Say When You Talk to Yourself by Shad Helmstetter, PhD

This is a book my fellow coaches and I often recommend. If you are serious about kicking that negative self-talk to the curb and you are ready to change into a more positive optimistic outlook, this is the book for you. I truly believe I was blessed to have a group of coaches who encouraged me to challenge my self-talk about my cancer and my future.

The Resilience Workbook: Essential Skills to Recover from Stress, Trauma, and Adversity by Glenn R. Schiraldi, PhD

Workbooks are great because they're full of actionable activities. I'm guessing every time you go to the doctor you will be asked about any overwhelming feelings of sadness or depression. Cancer certainly isn't a picnic. Take charge of your mental health with the tools you picked up in *Becoming Ovary Jones*, and take it to the next level with workbooks like this one. I particularly appreciated the chapter on Expressive Writing.

Toxin Toxout: Getting Harmful Chemicals Out of Our Bodies and Our World by Bruce Lourie and Rick Smith

This is the book that opened my eyes to a whole toxic world that I had been frolicking in my whole life. Something in our environment triggered our cancer. More and more people are being diagnosed every day. It might be wise to look at the world around us, and this book provides astonishing insight.

Want to learn more about faith? Honestly, *The Bible* is my go-to in this department. A few years ago, I asked one of my clients, "What is one thing you've been wanting to do but, for whatever reason, you just haven't made it happen?" Without hesitation, he told me he's been wanting to go to church. We had a brief discussion about that, and he decided by our next coaching session he would go to church.

On our next call he told me he dragged his feet for the whole two weeks, unable to muster up the courage each Sunday to cross that threshold. He said he knew I would be asking about it, so he made it happen the Wednesday night before our Thursday call. He's been going ever since.

A lot of people view their cancer as a wake-up call and an opportunity to make some big changes in their life. Perhaps you are ready for God. I'm sure there's a local church waiting for you to step inside.

APPENDIX B

PRACTICAL TIPS AND IDEAS

Some of your fellow Ovary Jones sisters wanted to give you a few tips nobody told us. Here's what we wish we would have known sooner.

HANDICAPPED PARKING

Every state is different, but we have found with a doctor's prescription and the Department of Motor Vehicles, you can get a placard for handicapped parking. You might not need it; however, the most common complaint of cancer patients is fatigue. If you need to pick up medicine at the pharmacy, it might help tremendously if you could park closer to the door. It is worth looking into it if you need it. Ask your doctor.

DAY PLANNER

Cancer is at least a part-time job. You will have a lot of appointments, tests, blood draws, and places to be. Organization is critical. Find a system that works for you to keep up with it. Ask help from friends or family.

PILL KEEPER

They now have pharmacies that will dispense your medicines into individual daily bags so there isn't any confusion. Personally, I can't use those because I have to get my medicine from a specialty pharmacy. The weekly or monthly pill containers are life savers. You will be asked at every appointment if you missed any doses. Have an organizational system for your pills so you can confidently say, "No." The drugs only work when you take them.

PRE-TREATMENT CHECKLIST

There are two types of people in the world: those who write lists and those who do not. Regardless of which category you fall into, keep a pre-chemo checklist if you are doing chemotherapy. (I wasn't a list person until I had to be.) Here are a few things you might want to include if they apply to you:

- Take your pre-meds (for nausea or anything else they suggest taking before treatment).

- Apply the numb cream if you have a port they will access. They will suggest when exactly to apply it.
- Wear a shirt that enables easy access to your port.
- Pack lunch and healthy snacks.
- Take a good book or something to occupy your time when you are awake.

DRINK PLENTY OF WATER

Vomiting, diarrhea, and the chemo drugs can cause you to get dehydrated, which further complicates things. This is something to talk to your team about if you are struggling.

NUTRITION IS CRITICAL

It's easy to become malnourished when you can't keep things down. Food might have a metallic or different taste also. Make it a priority to find foods you can eat. Choose a nutritionist for your team.

KEEP A FOOD, GRATITUDE, WELLNESS, AND RECOVERY JOURNAL

This is a time for tracking. Record how you are feeling each day, including your emotions and any symptoms or side effects. Pay attention to the time of day as well as how many days post-therapy you start feeling any adverse effects.

ASK QUESTIONS

As you go through this journey, you will feel like you should get a degree of some sort because you will learn so much. Ask all the questions you have. Keep a going list in your journal to take with you to your appointments so you don't forget to ask. Ask about the medicines they are giving you. Know the dosage of the things you take at home. If you are uncomfortable with a prescription, ask if there is anything else you could take. (Beth was prescribed something for tingling she was feeling in her feet. She didn't like it, so she asked if there was an alternative. For her, they told her to take Vitamin B3, and the tingling went away.) This is your recovery, and you are ultimately responsible for the decisions made in your treatment plan, including pharmacological agents.

MOVE WHEN YOU CAN

Yes, it sounds challenging. You want to try to maintain your muscle strength as much as possible. Even if you can't move your whole body (because you are in a wheelchair or something), try doing some arm raises. Anything you can do will help. Of course, listen to your doctors, but usually they recommend trying to move because, as counterproductive as it sounds, moving helps ease fatigue.

MEDICATE BEFORE SYMPTOMS

When advised, try to take the medicines they tell you to take to alleviate nausea, diarrhea/constipation, or pain before the symptoms knock you down. Listen to your doctors and stay ahead of the game as much as possible. This is where your journaling really pays off because you can look back to your previous treatment and see how you were feeling on the days that followed. It pays to pay attention.

ABUNDANT LIP BALM

Keep lip balm and lotion everywhere so you always have access to it.

GO TO A THERAPIST OR COUNSELOR

You are going through a lot, and your mental health is critical to your recovery. Make sure you have somebody on your team whom you can talk to about your feelings. Depression, mood swings, loneliness, and all kinds of thoughts and emotions are important to recognize. We can't pretend they don't exist. Get help processing it all. Honestly, I think everybody would benefit from therapy even if they don't have cancer.

WASH YOUR HANDS (A LOT)

Proper hand hygiene is always important, but now more than ever, you want to protect yourself. Along with all the obvious times to wash your hands, add before and after touching your medication.

DON'T BE TOUCHY

Avoid touching the germ poles on trams and subways and handrails on escalators and steps whenever possible. Your immune system is compromised, so you want to take some added precautions.

ASK FOR HELP

Cleaning, planning and preparing meals, walking the dog, taking care of children, driving to appointments, and other responsibilities could get challenging. Let people help you. If they don't volunteer, ask. (Don't create a story in your head as to why they didn't offer—this cancer diagnosis is new to them too.) You've most likely been helping people your whole life. It is perfectly acceptable, understandable, and reasonable to accept some help now.

SAY NO

Fighting cancer is your number-one, top priority right now. We tend to be busy people, and overcommitting is an easy pitfall to succumb to. Learn to say no, and take the time you need to plan your days.

GIVE YOURSELF PERMISSION TO HEAL

This is a process. It takes time. Allow yourself the grace you need to work your recovery plan. Listen to your body.

LEARN TECHNIQUES TO REDUCE STRESS

Consider this an opportunity to take up meditation or learn other ways to manage stress. Our bodies are not designed for chronic stress. The diagnosis and all the cancer talk can be a lot to take in.

ADOPT CHANGE

Perhaps there are things in your life you have been meaning to change. Many Ovary Jones sisters say this was the wake-up call they needed to change some things up. You can do it!

DELETE FRIENDS ON SOCIAL MEDIA

You can fire whomever you want to on social media, and usually they don't even know it. Surround yourself with positivity even online.

HAVE AN EXIT LINE

When you get sucked into a conversation with somebody that turns into them telling you a story about somebody they knew or it's just not uplifting you in general, politely excuse yourself from the conversation and bolt. We have to protect our minds, now more than ever.

ABOUT THE AUTHOR

MELANIE HOLSCHER is a high-performance leadership and business development coach passionate about lifting people up and helping them push beyond their belief barriers to strengthen their mental game and accomplish their goals. It's so gratifying when clients achieve results and reach echelons previously beyond their grasp, according to Melanie. Then Melanie was called to war on an unfamiliar battleground. Using skills usually applied to business and sports, Melanie fought cancer. Her bleak, Stage 4 Metastatic Ovarian Cancer diagnosis took her from the board room to a hospital room immediately. There she had to tap into her circle of influence—other coaches from around the world—and hammer out the ultimate mental game with the highest stakes at risk. Grateful for every miraculous day as a survivor, Melanie's mission is to create a movement to change the way the cancer battle is fought by strengthening the mental game. "We have to win in our mind before we can start the fight in our body," says Melanie.

Melanie and her daughter and social media consultant, Mackenzie Holscher, are founders of *Together We Box*, a monthly subscription box for cancer patients full of encouragement, gifts, and actionable hope. Fighting cancer is a marathon. Usually the people who love us want to help, but life is busy and the journey is long. The boxes are meant to be a power surge for warriors every month throughout the cancer battle. The boxes are packed with resilience, grit, and courage, and they are full of inspiration and encouragement. There is hope in every box and things for warriors to do to consistently toughen their mental game.

With a servant's heart, Melanie engages with audiences all over the world challenging their perception of adversity. Speaking at company sales meetings and leadership events and in churches, Melanie's inspiring message of actionable hope puts you in the driver's seat...of your career, of your health, and of your life.

JOIN THE MOVEMENT

Are you interested in having Melanie address your organization? Connect with Melanie or the *Together We Box* fight crew:

www.TogetherWeBox.com

Email: mackenzie@togetherwebox.com

Connect on LinkedIn: https://www.linkedin.com/in/mdholscher

CPSIA information can be obtained
at www.ICGtesting.com
Printed in the USA
LVHW030745301120
672994LV00018B/488/J